HIKING KENTUCKY'S
RED RIVER
GORGE
2nd Edition

SEAN PATRICK HILL

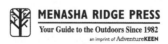

MENASHA RIDGE PRESS
Your Guide to the Outdoors Since 1982
an imprint of Adventure**KEEN**

Hiking Kentucky's Red River Gorge: Your Definitive Guide to the Jewel of the Southeast

Copyright © 2012 and 2019 by Sean Patrick Hill
All rights reserved
Published by Menasha Ridge Press
Distributed by Publishers Group West
Printed in China
Second edition, third printing 2022

Cover design and maps: Scott McGrew
Interior design: Annie Long
Cover photos: *Top:* Patrick Jennings/Shutterstock.com; *bottom:* Alexey Stiop/Shutterstock.com
Interior photos: Sean Patrick Hill
Project editor: Holly Cross
Proofreader: Emily Beaumont
Indexer: Rich Carlson

Library of Congress Cataloging-in-Publication Data
Names: Hill, Sean Patrick, author.
Title: Hiking Kentucky's Red River Gorge : your definitive guide to the jewel of the Southeast /
Sean Hill.
Description: Second edition. | Birmingham : Menasha Ridge Press, [2019]
Summary: "The rugged wilderness of Kentucky's Red River Gorge is like no other.
Dense forests, wondrous rock formations, and awe-inspiring views make it a paradise that's
waiting to be explored. Whether you're a beginner or an experienced hiker, you'll find carefully
maintained trails that are perfect for your needs"— Provided by publisher.
Identifiers: LCCN 2019018570 | ISBN 9781634041379 (paperback)
ISBN 9781634041386 (ebook)
Subjects: LCSH: Hiking—Kentucky—Red River Gorge—Guidebooks.
Red River Gorge (Ky.)—Guidebooks.
Classification: LCC GV199.42.K42 H55 2019 | DDC 796.5109769—dc23
LC record available at https://lccn.loc.gov/2019018570

 MENASHA RIDGE PRESS
An imprint of AdventureKEEN
2204 First Ave. S., Ste. 102
Birmingham, AL 35233
800-678-7006, fax 877-374-9016

Visit menasharidge.com for a complete listing of our books and for ordering information.
Contact us at our website, at facebook.com/menasharidge, or at twitter.com/menasharidge
with questions or comments. To find out more about who we are and what we're doing, visit
blog.menasharidge.com.

DISCLAIMER This book is intended only as a guide to select trails in the Red River Gorge area
and does not guarantee hiker safety—you hike at your own risk. Neither Menasha Ridge Press
nor Sean Patrick Hill is liable for property loss or damage, personal injury, or death that may
result from accessing or hiking the trails described. Please be especially cautious when walking in
potentially hazardous terrains with, for example, steep inclines or drop-offs. Please read carefully
the introduction to this book, as well as safety information from other sources. Familiarize
yourself with current weather reports and maps of the area you plan to visit (in addition to the
maps provided in this guidebook). Be cognizant of park regulations and always follow them. Do
not take chances.

OPPOSITE: VIEW FROM TUNNEL RIDGE ROAD

Dedication

For my daughter, Teagan; my brother, Michael; and everyone who bought my book the first time around.

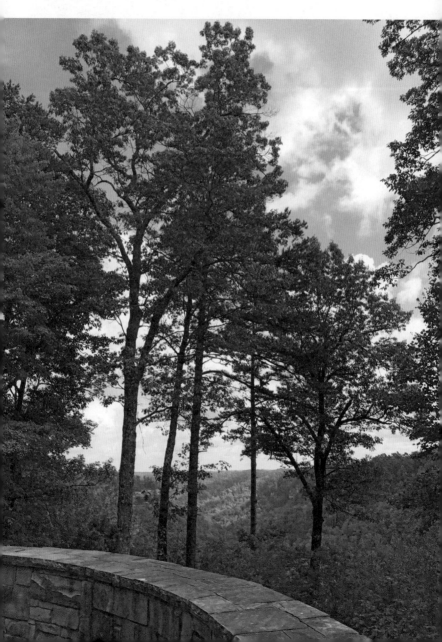

Hiking the Red River Gorge

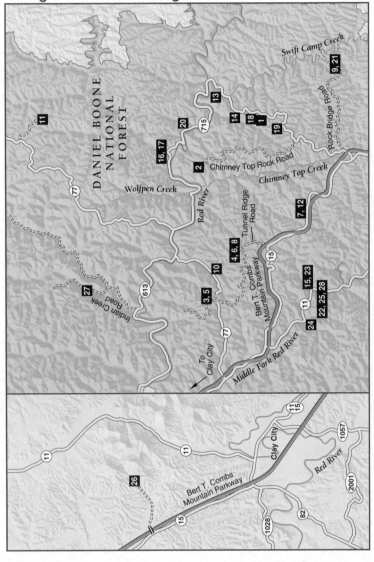

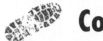

Contents

DEDICATION iii

OVERVIEW MAP opposite page

MAP LEGEND vii

ACKNOWLEDGMENTS viii

PREFACE ix

RECOMMENDED HIKES xi

INTRODUCTION 1

Red River Gorge Geological Area 31

1 Angel Windows 32

2 Chimney Top Rock, Princess Arch,
and Half Moon Arch 36

3 Courthouse Rock and Auxier Ridge 41

4 D. Boon Hut 46

5 Double Arch 50

6 Grays Arch 55

7 Koomer Ridge and Hidden Arch 59

8 Pinch-Em-Tight Ridge 64

9 Rock Bridge Arch 68

10 Rough Trail 73

11 Sheltowee Trace 79

12 Silvermine Arch and Cliff Trail 85

13 Sky Bridge 90

14 Whistling Arch 94

15 Whittleton Arch 98

Clifty Wilderness 104

16 Sheltowee Trace–Bison Way Loop 105

17 Sheltowee Trace–Osborne Bend Loop 110

18 Swift Camp Creek Trail 115

19 Swift Camp Creek–Wildcat Loop 121

20 Tower Rock 127

21 Turtle Back Arch 131

Natural Bridge State Resort Park   136

22 Balanced Rock and Rock Garden Trail 137

23 Henson's Cave Arch 142

24 Hood's Branch–Sand Gap Loop 147

25 The Original Trail 153

More Trails in the Red River Gorge Area   158

26 Pilot Knob State Nature Preserve 159

27 Powdermill Branch Trail. 163

28 White's Branch Arch 168

Appendixes and Index   173

APPENDIX A: OUTDOOR RETAILERS   174

APPENDIX B: HIKING CLUBS   176

APPENDIX C: STATE AND FEDERAL AGENCIES   177

INDEX   179

ABOUT THE AUTHOR   187

————	••••••••••••	··············
Featured trail	Alternate trail	Alternate trail
⬤━━━⬤	⊂═══⬤══⊃	⊂━━━⊃
Freeway	Highway with bridge	Minor road
================	•━•━•━•━•	
Unpaved road	Power line	

▭	🬀🬀🬀	～～～
Park/forest	Water body	River/creek/ intermittent stream

⌐ Bench	⑦ Information kiosk	⬩ Scenic view/overlook
△ Campground	🅿 Parking	⊏ Shelter
✕ Footbridge	▲ Peak/summit	🏯 Sheltowee Trace
•━• Gate	🎋 Picnic area	🧍 Trailhead
● General point of interest	🚻 Restroom	⌒ Tunnel (road)

Acknowledgments

I AM GRATEFUL for the many organizations and individuals who helped, whether they knew it or not, with the writing, hiking, and research necessary for this book:

Claire Suer, Susan Haynes, Holly Cross, Scott McGrew, and Emily Beaumont at Menasha Ridge Press, for their patience as I put together the book.

The staff at the Gladie Cultural-Environmental Learning Center in the Red River Gorge, for information and conditions on the trails.

Charlie Rowe, U.S. Forest Service employee and leader of the all-volunteer Red River Gorge Trail Crew, for some general updates on trails that had been updated or rerouted since this book's first edition.

Red River Gorgeous Cabin Rental for the use of the Huckleberry Farmhouse while I completed the last few hikes and photographs for this new edition.

The various authors who gave me the inspiration to start on the best hikes of the Gorge, including Wendell Berry, Jerrell Goodpaster, Robert Ruchhoft, Michael Brown, Hiram Rogers, and members of the Bluegrass Group of the Kentucky Sierra Club.

—Sean Patrick Hill

Preface

IT IS NOT UNWARRANTED to say that the preservation of Kentucky's Red River Gorge began with a single hike. More than 50 years ago, on November 18, 1967, members of the Cumberland Chapter of the Sierra Club invited U.S. Supreme Court Justice William O. Douglas for a walk in an area that, in the prevailing plan at the time, was to be flooded behind a dam. Joined by residents of the area who also opposed the dam, the group—which included a young Diane Sawyer, a correspondent from *The New York Times,* and hundreds of demonstrators—set out on a 3-mile hike in the wilderness along what is now a National Wild and Scenic River.

The plan would have called for the U.S. Army Corps of Engineers to build a dam to control flooding in the rolling countryside downstream from the Gorge. It helped that Justice Douglas was an avid environmentalist, calling places like the Gorge the "spiritual inheritance of America," as Lexington's *Herald-Leader* quoted him in its Sunday edition. Later, at a dinner hosted by the Sierra Club, Douglas told some 246 people that "We don't live, my friends, by bread alone; we live by the great spiritual values. That's why I think your fight for the little Red River Gorge is symbolic of the great fight that's going on all round the United States." This marks the Red River Gorge—which I would not say is "small" by any measure—as not only an impressive natural area but also as a legacy, much in the way that Yosemite National Park is a legacy bequeathed to the United States because Sierra Club founder John Muir had the foresight to invite then-President Teddy Roosevelt for a camping trip.

Still, it took time for the Gorge to be preserved as the national geologic area it is today. Public sentiment against the proposed dam grew, fueled in part by Wendell Berry's seminal book, *The Unforeseen Wilderness.* Eventually, the Army Corps of Engineers gave up. Today, the area sees about half a million visitors who hike, camp, rock climb, or just tour the well-paved loop in their automobiles. If the Gorge had not been preserved, many of the cliffs, rock shelters, and spectacular arches would have been submerged and lost.

When you first visit Red River Gorge, especially if you arrive from the Bluegrass region or the plains of Ohio, you almost immediately notice the landscape changing. The Red River carves its way out of the Cumberland Plateau, the uplifted striations of Newman limestone and iron-rich Corbin sandstone, rocks dating to the Mississippian and Pennsylvanian geologic periods, each more than 300 million years old. In spring, flowering rhododendron and pink lady's slippers adorn the stone; in autumn, the fiery leaves of red maple and the golden leaves of yellow poplar provide the palette. In winter, the cliffs are draped with ice, and in summer, with willowy maidenhair ferns.

Approaching the Gorge, you will undoubtedly have heard about its arches. Red River Gorge lays claim to the highest concentration of sandstone arches east of the Mississippi. Other arches are fashioned of limestone. Red River Gorge also has an incredible concentration of trees of an astounding variety—pine, maple, oak, magnolia, poplar, ash, beech, hickory, and hemlock. The Daniel Boone National Forest, of which the Gorge is a part, provides habitat for an estimated 67 different species of reptiles and amphibians, 46 species of mammals, and 100 species of birds, including Kentucky's famous warblers.

It bears repeating that because of the nature of the so-called soft rock present in Red River Gorge, in the next few million years the Red River will eventually carve a bed deeper than the Grand Canyon.

There are plenty of reasons to hike the Red River Gorge: exercise, sightseeing, bird-watching, backpacking, and more. I am of a mind that it is just as important to experience the Gorge as an emblem of the passage of time and the incredible forces of nature that have shaped it. This is what makes me agree with Justice Douglas that the Gorge is, in fact, a spiritual place. Though the Gorge is increasingly busy during warm weather, there is still an opportunity to find silence. That silence, not unlike the rock faces, the endangered species, and the pristine waterways of the Gorge, is well worth protecting.

Recommended Hikes

Best Hikes for Arches

  5 Double Arch (p. 50)

  6 Grays Arch (p. 55)

  9 Rock Bridge Arch (p. 68)

  13 Sky Bridge (p. 90)

  15 Whittleton Arch (p. 98)

  28 White's Branch Arch (p. 168)

Best Hikes for Backpacking

  11 Sheltowee Trace (p. 79)

  18 Swift Camp Creek Trail (p. 115)

Best Hikes for Geology

  1 Angel Windows (p. 32)

  4 D. Boon Hut (p. 46)

  22 Balanced Rock and Rock Garden Trail (p. 137)

Best Hikes for Kids

  2 Chimney Top Rock and Princess Arch (p. 36) (*Note:* Half Moon Arch, in the same hike profile, is too risky for children.)

  15 Whittleton Arch (p. 98)

  20 Tower Rock (p. 127)

  23 Henson's Cave Arch (p. 142)

  25 The Original Trail (p. 153)

Best Hikes for Scenic Creeks

  10 Rough Trail (p. 73)

  19 Swift Camp Creek–Wildcat Loop (p. 121)

Best Hikes for Seclusion

  17 Sheltowee Trace–Osborne Bend Loop (p. 110)

  21 Turtle Back Arch (p. 131)

  24 Hood's Branch–Sand Gap Loop (p. 147)

Best Hikes for Views

3   Courthouse Rock and Auxier Ridge (p. 41)

10   Rough Trail (p. 73)

16   Sheltowee Trace–Bison Way Loop (p. 105)

Best Hikes for Wildflowers

7   Koomer Ridge and Hidden Arch (p. 59)

VIRGINIA PINES OVERLOOK THE BLUEGRASS REGION. *(Hike 26, Pilot Knob State Nature Preserve, page 159)*

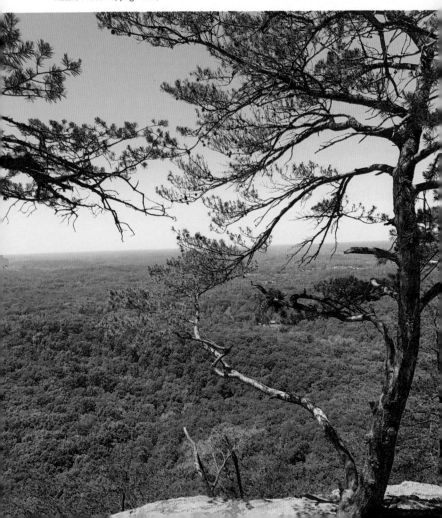

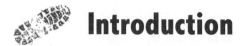 # Introduction

About This Book

Red River Gorge is a bit of a misnomer, as the bulk of the area described in this book encompasses three major geographic areas: Red River Gorge Geological Area, the Clifty Wilderness, and Natural Bridge State Resort Park. These three bordering areas together constitute what Kentuckians generally refer to as The Gorge.

Still another level of confusion arises from the fact that the actual gorge of the Red River composes only a small portion of the region. Further, the river has two branches—one running east to west through the Clifty Wilderness and into the geological area, and the other running through Natural Bridge State Resort Park. Generally, when people speak of *the* Red River, they mean the main branch of the river on U.S. Forest Service land. This is the river famous for canoeing and kayaking, sometimes perilously so. The funny thing is that with all the trail mileage one can rack up in the Red River Gorge, less than a mile of that is actually along the Red River itself; the Sheltowee Trace is the only trail that crosses it, and that on a justifiably famous suspension bridge.

Most of the hiking lies in the area around the Red River, especially to the south. That said, the entire Red River Gorge Geological Area is in fact a series of gorges or, more precisely, ravines. The Red River is fed by a number of branches that cut swaths through the surrounding countryside, which is on the western edge of the Cumberland Plateau. Thus, the Gorge has two major kinds of trails—ones that follow the creeks and bottomlands, alternately known as coves or hollows, and ones that follow the high ridgelines. Of course, there are the in-between trails as well—that is, the trails that climb to the ridges and descend to the creeks.

Every part of the Red River Gorge shares some commonalities. The famous arches, as well as the rock shelters, are present on both

U.S. Forest Service land and state-park property. Not all of them are clearly indicated on maps, either. But as far as the amazing rock formations go, they can be found in any part of the area.

The forests, too, vary by elevation but are consistent throughout the region. The lower-elevation mixed mesophytic forests are lush and dense, laden with both hardwood and conifer trees—including tulip poplars, mountain maples, eastern hemlocks, and bigleaf magnolias—and an understory of ferns and rhododendrons. The higher-elevation forests, those running along the ridges, tend to be drier, composed of tall oaks and pines intermixed with mountain laurels and blueberry brambles.

It can be argued that the real draw of the Red River Gorge, though, is the rock. With the most rock arches east of the Mississippi River, this area stands alone for scenery. Some of the spans, including Grays Arch and Natural Bridge, are justifiably crowd-drawing. But many other arches in the area that are easily accessible by trail—including Indian Arch, Double Arch, Silvermine Arch, and Whittleton Arch, to name a few—may not see quite as many visitors. The rock shelters, some of which have been used historically not only by Native Americans but also early settlers making gunpowder, are another vivid demonstration of nature's weathering powers. Finally, there are the cliffs and towering rock formations, many of which draw legions of rock climbers intent on tackling the nearly vertical walls.

This brings us to one of the most important aspects of the Red River Gorge: It is dangerous. The last few years have seen several deaths in the Gorge. I cannot overstate the perils inherent in the Gorge, especially around the arches and cliffs. Of the more pernicious reasons that the Gorge is famous, one is the death toll associated with people, especially young people, falling from the cliffs. Drop-offs can be abrupt, and in places where undergrowth obscures edges, disaster lurks. I also cannot overemphasize the need to take special care when hiking the Red River Gorge: *stay away from cliffs, and do not climb on arches.* Even trails can be perilous, especially in wet or icy weather—sandstone, in particular, is prone to becoming slippery with any degree of water.

Another issue with the rocks—with the Gorge in general—is their susceptibility of being loved to death. Indeed, since the region was saved from being flooded by a proposed dam back in the 1960s, the area has only gained in reputation. With the frequency of visitors—and on summer days, this is readily apparent—comes increased damage. Everywhere in the Gorge there are carvings left by people, the occasional historical petroglyph notwithstanding. Trash is evident throughout the area as well, as are the overly used and often illegal campsites, which crowd along the creeks and trails to the point that hikers will often encounter a roped-off plot where the U.S. Forest Service has closed a decrepit site to allow for its recovery. It is important to follow Leave No Trace guidelines here, as with anywhere.

That said, you can carve out a niche for yourself here without carving your name into the rock. Many times of year, if not midweek in summer, you can have a large swath of wilderness to yourself. Sure, some portions of the Gorge are crowded, making parking an exercise in patience, but many more sections are empty. The Clifty Wilderness, for one, is a great place to backpack, with plenty of spots that follow federal regulations and allow for low-impact camping.

Also consider that the most popular times to go can also be more troublesome. Spring, while it brings the rare Kentucky wildflowers, also means high water, especially on larger creeks that may become simply impassable. Summer often means humidity and heat and an impressive array of insects, though not always. With its fireworks display of changing leaves, autumn makes the Gorge famous. October is the best and, maybe unfortunately, most popular time to visit. Backpacking and rock climbing are heaviest at this time. Still, consider going early in the day or bypassing the popular spots. Head for the hills instead.

Late fall and winter are surprisingly wonderful times to experience the Gorge. For one thing, the weather and temperature are sometimes perfect. Second, when the leaves come down, the starkness of the cliffs and rock formations—what you may never have noticed in the depths of summer—are readily apparent. The views open, and crowds on the trail thin. The main concern at this time is ice, which happens virtually anywhere there is a cliff—limestone, for one, is essentially porous by nature, and the water that gushes through its cracks freezes, forming both incredible ice waterfalls and dangerously slick trails.

For the ambitious, especially those considering long backpacking treks, it's important to note that the Sheltowee Trace, Kentucky's most famous trail, traverses north to south through most of the areas presented in this guide. This 300-plus-mile trail enters the Clifty Wilderness at the end of Corner Ridge Road, then traverses the Red River Gorge Geological Area, crossing the Red River and continuing to the Whittleton Campground: 17 miles in all. From there, the Trace continues another 5 miles through Natural Bridge State Resort Park. Easily identifiable by the white turtle blazes (*Sheltowee*, the name given by the Shawnee natives to Daniel Boone, means "turtle"), the Trace offers not only a continuous hike through the Gorge but also serves as an important connector to a number of other trails.

The Rough Trail is the other significant trail, as it crosses east to west the length of Red River Gorge Geological Area and is, in my opinion, the single best hike in the Gorge. Topping ridge after ridge, descending and descending again to lovely creeks, this single 7.7-mile hike offers the best views and some of the best backpacking spots.

The hikes detailed in this book cover every major trail in the Red River Gorge. They are arranged in numerous fashions, allowing for day hikes of varying lengths, times, and difficulties, some out-and-backs, and some loops. For the most part, if you undertake all of these hikes, you will have seen the best the Gorge has to offer. I chose hikes not only for the value of destinations, such as arches, but also for exploration of the various topography of the Gorge. Despite the seeming brevity of some treks, all are worth experiencing.

Although the Gorge may seem imposing at times, don't let that stop you. Yes, the Gorge has its risks, but for the conscientious hiker, the rewards far outnumber the dangers. Remember to stay safe, and it's likely that you'll meet good souls on the trail willing to share a secret or two. For me, it was a couple of guys on the Whittleton Branch Trail; they told me to watch for the slats of wood lining the trail in a boggy section. These, I was told, were the original ties for the old logging railroad that ran here. How could I have known that? Then they told me how to find a secret rock shelter just on the other side of a hidden waterfall. You get the picture.

It really takes only one good hike to fall in love with the Red River Gorge. After that, you'll find yourself thinking about it again and again.

ANGEL WINDOWS IS A GREAT SPOT TO STOP FOR LUNCH WHILE EXPLORING.
(Hike 1, page 32)

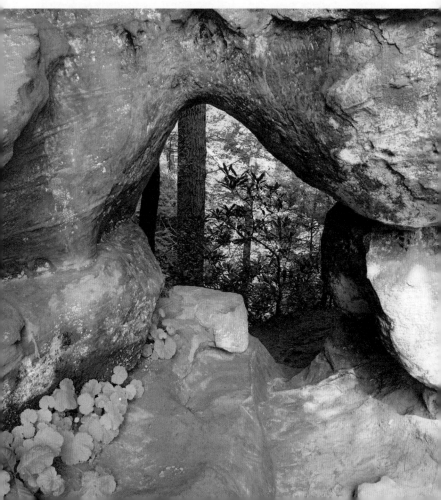

Red River Gorge Geological Area

One of the crown jewels of the Daniel Boone National Forest, and of Kentucky as a whole, is this 29,000-acre expanse. First designated as a geological area by the U.S. Forest Service in 1974, the Red River Gorge was also named a National Natural Landmark by the National Park Service in 1976. A full 19.4 miles of the Red River are designated as a National Wild and Scenic River, the first in Kentucky, with 46 miles of roadway designated a National Scenic Byway—much of this route being the main access to the trails that thread this area.

More than 100 natural arches dot the region, not to mention the rock shelters, steep cliffs, and occasional cave. Mostly composed of sedimentary stone, the Red River Gorge area was formed some 300 million years ago as the ancient Appalachian Mountains were eroded by a vast river and deposited along the shore of the now extinct inland sea that covered much of what is now North America. Over time, this sediment became stone and was lifted and carved by water and wind into what is now a landscape as diverse in topography as it is in plants and animals. Sweet birch and yellow buckeye exist in the same spaces as white-haired goldenrod—a threatened species found nowhere else in the world.

The bulk of the trails in Red River Gorge are found in the geological area. Opportunities for backpacking, day hikes, and short strolls abound. Car camping is also an option, so long as you purchase the required overnight permit and pitch your tent at least 300 feet from any U.S. Forest Service road. The sole public camping area in Red River Gorge is Koomer Ridge Campground, with 54 first-come, first-served sites equipped with picnic tables, lantern posts, and plenty of space. The campground also has a bathhouse, drinking water, and vault toilets, as well as direct access to a number of trails.

Some of the numerous sites of note in the geological area are Grays Arch, the largest in the Gorge, as well as Courthouse Rock, Double Arch, the Rough Trail, Sky Bridge, the Chimney Top Rock viewpoint, and many more. Three state highways—KY 15, KY 77, and KY 715—compose the scenic byway, forming a loop around the geological area and the Red River itself.

Clifty Wilderness

In 1985 the Kentucky Wilderness Act passed by Congress designated nearly half of the geological area as the Clifty Wilderness, one of only two wilderness areas in the state. At 12,646 acres, it is a substantial plot of land that, surprisingly, hosts only a few trails in its 20 square miles, including part of the Sheltowee Trace, the Osborne Bend Loop, and the Swift Camp Creek and Wildcat Trails. But all told, there are 20 miles of trail.

The Clifty certainly has the character of a wilderness. The trails are not nearly as maintained as those in the neighboring geological area, and they are decidedly less used. In that regard, the area can be rugged, but this allows for a profound sense of solitude; encountering other hikers can be an infrequent event. Excepting busy times, you'll find far more opportunities for backpacking spots in the Clifty than in the nearby geological area.

Part of the attraction to the Clifty Wilderness is the water. Some of the largest creeks in the region flow here, including Swift Camp Creek and the upper reaches of Gladie Creek, both of which are fed by numerous branches. Swift Camp Creek carves itself a narrow notch known as Hell's Kitchen, and Gladie twists languidly among boulders strewn with rhododendron blooms, like something out of an ancient Chinese painting. Both creeks are wide, and one need only cross them to find the true expanse of wilderness, as well as prime territory for tent pitching.

Because of the lack of trail maintenance and use, expect a lot of spiderwebs across your face, not to mention some eroded trails. But what the wilderness lacks in ease it makes up for in adventure: even a simple trek, such as that to Turtle Back Arch, can seem adventurous, with its cliff-scaling and abandoned-road route-finding.

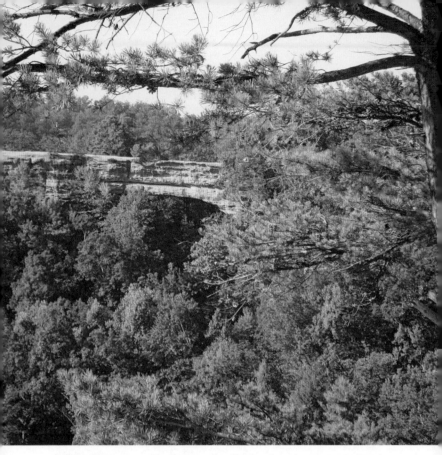

NATURAL BRIDGE IS ONE OF KENTUCKY'S MOST-VISITED NATURAL WONDERS.

Natural Bridge State Resort Park

One of the best and most popular state parks in Kentucky, Natural Bridge can be one of the busiest places in the Gorge—if not the state. With a lodge, restaurant, sky lift, several campgrounds, and, of course, the main attraction of Natural Bridge (the Gorge's second-biggest arch behind nearby Grays Arch), this area sees quite a few footprints. It's no surprise then that the trail that leads most directly to the arch, The Original Trail, built by the railroad company that hauled lumber out of the Gorge in the last century, is as wide as a road and maintained as such.

Some hard-core hikers forgo the state park, but I am not among them. Natural Bridge has an abundance of sights, a real sense of solitude, and, let's face it, one of the most difficult hikes in the entire Gorge. The Middle Fork of the Red River flows through the park but is not at all the attraction. Balanced Rock, the Rock Garden, and Laurel Ridge are attractions, though, and the stretch of the Sheltowee Trace that passes through the park leads up flight after flight of stairs as it soars to a large gazebo at Natural Bridge. In fact, there are many shelters throughout the park, built in the 1930s by the Civilian Conservation Corps.

Hitting the trails early or midweek is a sure way to avoid crowds. It is possible to stand atop Natural Bridge or at the famed lookout on Laurel Ridge and watch the sunrise with nary a human about. The other way to achieve solitude here is to realize that Natural Bridge and Laurel Ridge divide the park into what could be accurately called front- and backcountry. The western side of the park is without a doubt backcountry, a vast wilderness where the trail signs are uninhibited in proclaiming the difficulty of, say, the Sand Gap Trail—a long, arduous hike that twists in and out of the upper reaches of the Hood Branch watershed.

Natural Bridge provides campgrounds, though of a different nature than those found on federal lands. Whittleton Campground, though small and dense, provides water, a bathhouse, and access to the Sheltowee Trace, a portion of which follows the campground's entrance road. The Sheltowee Trace also provides access to the state park trails via Balanced Rock Trail and access to the geological area trails via Whittleton Branch Trail. It's worth your while to spend a few days at the campground and explore all the trails in the park.

How To Use This Guidebook

The following information walks you through this guidebook's organization to make it easy and convenient to plan great hikes.

Overview Map and Map Legend

The overview map on page iv shows the location of the primary trailheads for all hikes in this book. Each hike's number appears on the overview map and in the table of contents facing the overview map.

As you flip through the book, a hike's full profile is easy to locate by watching for the hike number at the top of each page. A map legend that details the symbols found on the trail maps appears on page vii.

Trail Maps

A detailed map of each hike's route appears with its profile. On each of these maps, symbols indicate the trailhead, the complete route, significant features, facilities, and topographic landmarks such as creeks, overlooks, and peaks.

To produce the highly accurate maps in this book, I used a handheld GPS unit to gather data while hiking each route and then sent that data to Menasha Ridge's expert cartographers. However, your GPS device is no substitute for sound, sensible navigation that takes into account the conditions that you observe while hiking.

Further, despite the high quality of the maps in this guidebook, the publisher and I strongly recommend that you always carry an additional map, such as the ones noted in each entry's listing for "Maps."

Elevation Profile

Each hike description's key info lists the elevation at the trailhead, as well as the elevation peak. That information is supplemented by a graphic illustration that represents the rises and falls of the trail as viewed from the side, over the complete mileage, of that trail. (One-way hikes are indicated with an arrow pointing right; out-and-backs are indicated with a double-ended arrow.) On the diagram's vertical axis, or height scale, the number of feet indicated between each tick mark lets you visualize the climb. To avoid making flat hikes look steep and steep hikes appear flat, varying height scales provide an accurate image of each hike's climbing challenge.

The Hike Profile

Each profile opens with the hike's star ratings, GPS trailhead coordinates, and other key at-a-glance information—from the trail's distance and configuration to contacts for local information. Each profile also includes a map (see "Trail Maps," page 10). The main text for each profile includes three sections: Overview, Route Details, and Directions (for driving to the trailhead area).

Star Ratings

Following is the explanation for the rating system of one to five stars in each of the five categories for each hike.

FOR SCENERY:

★★★★★	Unique, picturesque panoramas
★★★★	Diverse vistas
★★★	Pleasant views
★★	Unchanging landscape
★	Not selected for scenery

FOR TRAIL CONDITION:

★★★★★	Consistently well maintained
★★★★	Stable, with no surprises
★★★	Average terrain to negotiate
★★	Inconsistent, with good and poor areas
★	Rocky, overgrown, or often muddy

FOR CHILDREN:

★★★★★	Babes in strollers are welcome
★★★★	Fun for anyone past the toddler stage
★★★	Good for young hikers with proven stamina
★★	Not enjoyable for children
★	Not advisable for children ·

FOR DIFFICULTY:

★★★★★	Grueling
★★★★	Strenuous
★★★	Moderate (won't beat you up—but you'll know you've been hiking)
★★	Easy with patches of moderate
★	Good for a relaxing stroll

FOR SOLITUDE:

★★★★★	Positively tranquil
★★★★	Spurts of isolation
★★★	Moderately secluded
★★	Crowded on weekends and holidays
★	Steady stream of individuals and/or groups

GPS Trailhead Coordinates

As noted in "Trail Maps," on page 10, I used a handheld GPS unit to obtain geographic data and sent the information to the publisher's cartographers. In the key info for each hike profile, the numerical coordinates—the intersection of latitude (north) and longitude (west)—will orient you from the trailhead. In some cases, you can drive within viewing distance of a trailhead. Other hiking routes require a short walk to the trailhead from a parking area.

The latitude–longitude grid system is likely already familiar to you, but here's a refresher. Imaginary lines of latitude—called *parallels* and approximately 69 miles apart from each other—run horizontally around the globe. The equator is established to be 0°, and each parallel is indicated by degrees from the equator: up to 90°N at the North Pole, and down to 90°S at the South Pole.

Imaginary lines of longitude—called *meridians*—run perpendicular to latitude lines. Longitude lines are likewise indicated by degrees. Starting from 0° at the Prime Meridian in Greenwich, England, they continue to the east and west until they meet 180° later at the International Date Line in the Pacific Ocean. At the equator, longitude lines also are approximately 69 miles apart, but that distance narrows as the meridians converge toward the North and South Poles.

This guidebook uses the degree–decimal minute format for presenting GPS coordinates. For example, the coordinates for Hike 1 (page 32) are N37° 47.932' W83° 35.473'. To convert GPS coordinates given in degrees, minutes, and seconds to degrees–decimal minutes, the seconds are divided by 60. For more on GPS technology, visit usgs.gov.

DISTANCE & CONFIGURATION

Distance notes the length of the hike round-trip, from start to finish. If the hike description includes options to shorten or extend the hike, those round-trip distances will also be factored here. *Configuration* defines the trail as a loop, a point-to-point, an out-and-back (taking you in and out via the same route), a figure eight, or a balloon.

HIKING TIME

Every hiker has a different pace, but 2–3 miles per hour is a general rule of thumb for the hiking times noted in this guidebook. That pace typically allows time for taking photos, dawdling and admiring views, and alternating between stretches of hills and descents. When deciding whether to follow a particular trail in this guidebook, consider your own pace, weather, general physical condition, and energy level on a given day.

HIGHLIGHTS

Waterfalls, historical sites, or other features that draw hikers to the trail are emphasized here.

ELEVATION

The elevation at the trailhead is listed, along with another figure for the highest or lowest altitude on the route. If there is no significant gain, that is also noted.

ACCESS

Trails in the Daniel Boone National Forest are accessible day and night, year-round. However, any vehicle parked on KY 15 or in any area in the Red River Gorge Geological Area and the Indian Creek area north of KY 15 must display a backcountry permit from 10 p.m. to 6 a.m. Permits are available at a number of vendors in the area and also at the Gladie Cultural-Environmental Learning Center or the district office. Cost is $3 a day, $5 for three days, and $30 for an annual pass. The Interagency Pass allows for a 50% discount.

Koomer Ridge Campground is open year-round, as is access to potable water and vault toilets. (Its bathhouse, with flush toilets and showers, is unavailable in winter.) Campsites are paid for on-site. April 15–October 31, walk-in sites cost $20, drive-in single sites are $25, and double sites are $30 (an extra vehicle costs $8 per night). November 1–April 14, all sites are $10. The Interagency Pass allows for a 50% discount.

MAPS

The best map for the area is the topographic Red River Gorge Geological Area map published by the Daniel Boone National Forest, priced at $20. The USGS topographic maps for the Red River Gorge area, including Natural Bridge State Resort Park, are *Slade* and *Pomeroyton.* As previously noted, the publisher and I recommend that you carry more than one map—and that you consult those maps before heading out on the trail in order to resolve any confusion or discrepancy.

FACILITIES

This section alerts you to restrooms, water, picnic tables, and other basics at or near the trailhead.

WHEELCHAIR ACCESS

At-a-glance, you'll see if there are paved sections or other areas for safely using a wheelchair. In general, the majority of the Red River Gorge area is not wheelchair-accessible, though there are a select few paved trails in the geological area and Natural Bridge State Resort Park.

COMMENTS

Here you will find assorted nuggets of information, such as whether dogs are allowed on the trails.

CONTACTS

Phone numbers and websites listed here are handy for checking trail conditions and gleaning other day-to-day information.

Overview, Route Details, and Directions

These three elements compose the heart of the hike description. "Overview" gives you a quick summary of what to expect on that trail; "Route Details" guides you on the hike, start to finish; and "Directions" will get you to the trailhead from a well-known road or highway.

Weather

Weather in the Red River Gorge can be fickle. In general, spring means melting snow and rain, which can lead to high creeks and muddy trails. Summer is notable, as it is throughout Kentucky, for its high humidity and occasional heat indexes that can make hiking uncomfortable, even dangerous. Autumn is by far the best time to be in the Gorge, with its abundant sunshine and mild temperatures. In winter, the Gorge is accessible, and temperatures can be agreeable, but the dominant issue at this time is ice and snow, which can prove hazardous on many trails.

The following table lists average temperatures and precipitation by month for the Red River Gorge region. For each month, "High" is the average daytime high, "Low" is the average nighttime low, and "Rain or Snow" is the average precipitation.

MONTH	HIGH	LOW	RAIN OR SNOW
January	42°F	19°F	3.46"
February	48°F	21°F	3.07"
March	58°F	29°F	4.02"
April	68°F	37°F	3.62"
May	76°F	46°F	4.84"
June	83°F	56°F	4.02"
July	87°F	61°F	5.08"
August	86°F	59°F	3.50"
September	70°F	51°F	3.11"
October	70°F	38°F	2.83"
November	58°F	30°F	3.31"
December	47°F	24°F	4.02"

Water

How much is enough? Well, one simple physiological fact should convince you to err on the side of excess when deciding how much water to pack: a hiker walking steadily in 90° heat needs approximately 10 quarts of fluid per day. That's 2.5 gallons. A good rule of thumb is to hydrate prior to your hike, carry (and drink) 6 ounces of water for every mile you plan to hike, and hydrate again after the hike. For most people, the pleasures of hiking make carrying water a relatively minor price to pay to remain safe and healthy. So pack more water than you anticipate needing, even for short hikes.

If you are tempted to drink "found water," do so with extreme caution. Many ponds and lakes are fairly stagnant, and the water tastes terrible. Drinking such water presents inherent risks for thirsty trekkers. Giardia parasites contaminate many water sources and cause the dreaded intestinal disorder giardiasis, which can last for weeks after onset. For more information, visit the Centers for Disease Control and Prevention website: cdc.gov/parasites/giardia.

In any case, effective treatment is essential before using any water source found along the trail. Boiling water for 2–3 minutes is always a safe measure for camping, but day hikers can consider iodine tablets, approved chemical mixes, filtration units rated for giardia, and UV filtration. Some of these methods (for example, filtration with an added carbon filter) remove bad tastes typical in stagnant water, while others add their own taste. Carry a means of water purification to help in a pinch and if you realize you have underestimated your consumption needs.

In the Red River Gorge, availability of drinkable water varies widely. Some trails follow high ridges where there is no water, while others follow or cross creeks or even pass springs. Note that as summer progresses, smaller water sources will begin to dry up.

Clothing

Factors such as weather, unexpected trail conditions, fatigue, hikes of extended duration, and wrong turns can individually or collectively turn a great outing into a very uncomfortable one at best—and a life-threatening one at worst. Thus, proper attire plays a key role in staying comfortable and, sometimes, in staying alive. Here are some helpful guidelines:

★ Choose silk, wool, or synthetics for maximum comfort in all of your hiking attire. Cotton is fine if the weather remains dry and stable, but you won't be happy if that material gets wet.

★ Always wear a hat, or at least tuck one into your day pack or hitch it to your belt. Hats offer all-weather sun and wind protection as well as warmth if it turns cold.

★ Be ready to layer up or down as the day progresses and the mercury rises or falls. Today's outdoor wear makes layering easy, with such designs as jackets that convert to vests and zip-off or button-up legs.

★ Wear hiking boots or sturdy hiking sandals with toe protection. Flip-flopping along a paved urban greenway is one thing, but never hike a trail in open sandals or casual sneakers. Your bones and arches need support, and your skin needs protection.

★ Pair that footwear with good socks. If you prefer not to sheathe your feet when wearing hiking sandals, tuck the socks into your day pack; you may need them if the weather plummets or if you hit rocky turf and pebbles begin to irritate your feet. And, in an emergency, if you have lost your gloves, you can adapt the socks into mittens.

★ Don't leave raingear behind, even if the day dawns clear and sunny. Tuck into your day pack, or tie around your waist, a jacket that is breathable and either water-resistant or waterproof. Investigate different choices at your local outdoors retailer. If you are a frequent hiker, ideally you'll have more than one raingear weight, material, and style in your closet to protect you in all seasons in your regional climate and hiking microclimates.

Essential Gear

Today you can buy outdoor vests that have up to 20 pockets shaped and sized to carry everything from toothpicks to binoculars. Or, if you don't aspire to feel like a burro, you can neatly stow all of these items in your day pack or backpack. The following list showcases never-hike-without-them items, in alphabetical order, as all are important:

★ *Extra food:* Trail mix, granola bars, or other high-energy snacks.

★ *Flashlight or headlamp* with extra bulb and batteries.

★ *Insect repellent:* For some areas and seasons, this is extremely vital.

★ *Maps and a high-quality compass:* Even if you know the terrain from previous hikes, don't leave home without these. And, as previously noted, bring maps in addition to those in this guidebook, and consult your maps prior to the hike. If you are versed in GPS usage, bring that device too; but don't rely on it as your sole navigational tool, as battery life can dwindle or die, and be sure to compare its guidance with that of your maps.

★ *Pocketknife and/or a multitool:* Never hike without one of these implements.

★ *Sunscreen:* Be sure to check the expiration date on the tube or bottle.

★ *Water:* As emphasized more than once, bring more than you think you'll drink. Depending on your destination, you may want to bring a container and iodine or a filter for purifying water in case you run out.

★ *Whistle:* It could become your best friend in an emergency.

★ *Windproof matches and/or a lighter:* A fire starter is also a good idea.

First Aid Kit

In addition to the items above, those below may appear overwhelming for a day hike. But any paramedic will tell you that the products listed here—in alphabetical order because all are important—are just the basics. The reality of hiking is that you can be out for a week of backpacking and acquire only a mosquito bite. Or you can hike for an hour, slip, and suffer a bleeding abrasion or broken bone. Fortunately, these items will collapse into a very small space, and convenient, pre-packaged kits are available at your pharmacy and on the internet.

★ Ace bandages or Spenco joint wraps

★ Adhesive bandages

★ Antibiotic ointment (Neosporin or the generic equivalent)

★ Athletic tape

★ Benadryl or the generic equivalent, diphenhydramine (in case of allergic reactions)

★ Blister kit (such as Moleskin/Spenco 2nd Skin)

★ Butterfly-closure bandages

★ Epinephrine in a prefilled syringe (typically by prescription only, and for people known to have severe allergic reactions to hiking mishaps such as bee stings)

★ Gauze (one roll and a half dozen 4-by-4-inch pads)

★ Hydrogen peroxide or iodine

★ Ibuprofen or acetaminophen

General Safety

Mother Nature has no sympathy for the foolish or unlucky. If you'll be journeying beyond sight of your car, take the following sensible precautions, which may have the familiar ring of mom's voice as you take note of them.

★ *Always let someone know where you will be hiking and how long you expect to be gone.* It's a good idea to give that person a copy of your route, particularly if you are headed into any isolated area. Let them know when you return.

★ *Always sign in and out of any trail registers provided.* Don't hesitate to comment on the trail condition if space is provided; that's your opportunity to alert others to any problems you encounter.

★ *Don't count on a cell phone for your safety.* Reception may be spotty or nonexistent on the trail, even on an urban walk—especially one that's embraced by towering trees.

★ *Always carry food and water, even for a short hike.* And bring more water than you think you will need. (I can't say this often enough!)

★ *Ask questions.* State-forest and state-park employees are there to help. It's a lot easier to solicit advice before a problem occurs, and it will help you avoid a mishap away from civilization when it's too late to amend an error.

★ *Stay on designated trails.* Even on the most clearly marked trails, there is usually a point where you have to stop and consider in which direction to head. If you become disoriented, don't panic. As soon as you think you may be off track, stop, assess your current direction, and then retrace your steps to the point where you went astray. Using a map, a compass, and this book, and keeping in mind what you have passed thus far, reorient yourself, and trust your judgment on which way to continue. If you become absolutely unsure of how to continue, return to your vehicle the way you came in. Should you become completely lost and have no idea how to find the trailhead, remaining in place along the trail and waiting for help is most often the best option for adults, and always the best option for children.

★ *Always carry a whistle,* another precaution that cannot be overemphasized. It may be a lifesaver if you do become lost or sustain an injury.

★ *Be especially careful when crossing streams.* Whether you are fording the stream or crossing on a log, make every step count. If you have any doubt about maintaining your balance on a log, ford the stream instead: use a trekking pole or stout stick for balance and face upstream as you cross. If a stream seems too deep to ford, turn back. Whatever is on the other side is not worth risking your life.

★ *Be careful at overlooks.* While these areas may provide spectacular views, they are potentially hazardous. Stay back from the edge of outcrops, and make absolutely sure of your footing; a misstep can mean a nasty and possibly fatal fall.

★ *Be aware that standing dead trees and storm-damaged living trees pose significant hazards to hikers.* These trees may have loose or broken limbs that could fall at any time. While walking beneath trees, and when choosing a spot to rest or enjoy your snack, look up!

★ *Know the symptoms of subnormal body temperature, or hypothermia.* Shivering and forgetfulness are the two most common indicators of this stealthy killer. Hypothermia can occur at any elevation, even in summer, especially when the hiker is wearing lightweight cotton clothing. If symptoms present themselves, get to shelter, hot liquids, and dry clothes as soon as possible.

★ *Likewise, know the symptoms of heat exhaustion, or hyperthermia.* Lightheadedness and loss of energy are the first two indicators. If you feel these symptoms, find shade, drink water, remove as many layers of clothing as practical, and stay put until you cool down. Marching through heat exhaustion leads to heatstroke, which can be fatal. If you should be sweating and you're not, that's the signature warning sign. Your hike is over at that point—heatstroke is a life-threatening condition that can cause seizures, convulsions, and eventually death. If you or a companion reaches that point, do whatever can be done to cool the victim down and seek medical attention immediately.

★ *Most important of all, take along your brain.* A cool, calculating mind is the single-most important asset on the trail. Think before you act. Watch your step. Plan ahead. Avoiding accidents before they happen is the best way to ensure a rewarding and relaxing hike.

Watchwords for Flora and Fauna

Hikers should remain aware of the following concerns regarding plant life and wildlife, described in alphabetical order.

BLACK BEARS Black bear populations are growing in eastern Kentucky. Though attacks by black bears are uncommon, the sight or approach of a bear can give anyone a start. If you encounter a bear while hiking, remain calm and avoid running in any direction. Make loud noises to scare off the bear and back away slowly. In primitive and remote areas, assume bears are present; in more-developed sites, check out the current bear situation prior to hiking. Most encounters are food-related, as bears have an exceptional sense of smell and not particularly discriminating tastes. While this is of greater concern to backpackers and campers, on a day hike, you may plan a lunchtime picnic or will munch on an energy bar or other snack from time to time. So remain aware and alert.

The federally managed portion of the Red River Gorge area enforces several prohibitions concerning food storage. You may not do the following:

★ Possess, store, or leave any food (including food for pets and livestock, except baled hay), refuse, or bear attractant unless it is a) properly stored in a bear-resistant container; b) suspended at least 10 feet clear of the ground at all points, suspended at least 4 feet horizontally from the supporting tree or pole, and suspended at least 4 feet from any other tree or pole adjacent to the supporting tree or pole; c) stored in a closed motor vehicle with a solid top; d) stored in a closed, hard-body trailer; or e) being eaten, being prepared for eating, or being transported.

★ Discard or abandon any food, refuse, or bear attractant unless it is a) disposed of in a bear-resistant trash receptacle or other receptacle that has been provided by the U.S. Forest Service specifically for that purpose.

★ Burn or bury any food, refuse, or bear attractant.

BLACK FLIES Though certainly a pest and maddening annoyance, the worst a black fly will cause is an itchy welt. They are most active from mid-May into June, during the day, and especially before thunderstorms, as well as during the morning and evening hours. Insect repellent has some effect, though the only way to keep out of their swarming midst is to keep moving.

MOSQUITOES Ward off these pests with insect repellent and/or repellent-impregnated clothing. In some areas, mosquitoes are known to carry the West Nile virus, so take care to avoid their bites.

POISON IVY & OAK Recognizing and avoiding these plants are the most effective ways to prevent the painful, itchy rashes associated with them. Poison ivy (see top right) is by far the problematic plant in the Red River Gorge and occurs as a vine or groundcover, three leaflets to a leaf; poison oak (see bottom right) occurs as either a vine or shrub, also with three leaflets. Urushiol, the oil in the sap of these plants, is responsible for the rash. Within 14 hours

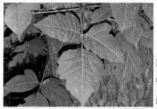

Photo: Tom Watson

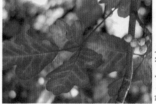
Photo: Jane Huber

of exposure, raised lines and/or blisters will appear on the affected area, accompanied by a terrible itch. Refrain from scratching, because bacteria under your fingernails can cause an infection. Wash and dry the affected area and apply calamine lotion to help dry out the rash. If itching or blistering is severe, seek medical attention. Remember that oil-contaminated clothes, hiking gear, and pets can easily cause an irritating rash on you or someone else, so wash them as necessary, along with any exposed parts of your body.

Poison ivy typically occurs near disturbed areas, such as the edges of trailhead parking lots and trailside. The most invasive areas are frequently closer to roads but not always.

SNAKES Rattlesnakes, cottonmouths, copperheads, and coral snakes are among the most common venomous snakes in the United States, and their hibernation season is typically October–April. In the region described in this book, you will possibly encounter the copperhead, the water moccasin, and the timber rattler (see below). However, the snakes you will most likely see while hiking will be nonvenomous species and subspecies. The best rule is to leave all snakes alone, give them a wide berth as you hike past, and make sure any hiking companions (including dogs) do the same.

Photo: Paul Staniszewski/ Shutterstock

When hiking, stick to well-used trails and wear over-the-ankle boots and loose-fitting long pants. Do not step or put your hands beyond your range of detailed visibility, and avoid wandering around in the dark. Step *onto* logs and rocks, never *over* them, and be especially careful when climbing rocks. Always avoid walking through dense brush or willow thickets.

STINGING NETTLES Frequent along trails throughout Kentucky, the common nettle is easy to avoid once you memorize what it looks like and, in the high summer periods, wear long pants. This plant is armed with tiny spicules that impale the skin and cause itching and burning. As with poison ivy, it thrives on disturbed ground.

TICKS These arachnids are often found on brush and tall grass, where they seem to be waiting to hitch a ride on a warm-blooded passerby. Adult ticks are most active April–May and again October–November. Among the varieties of ticks, the black-legged tick, commonly called the deer tick, is the primary carrier of Lyme disease. Wear light-colored clothing, which makes it easier for you to spot ticks before they migrate to your skin. At the end of your hike, visually check your hair, back of neck, armpits, and socks. During your posthike shower, take a moment to do a more complete body check. For ticks that are already embedded, removal with tweezers is best. Use disinfectant solution on the wound.

VIRGINIA BIG-EARED BATS In recent years, North American bats have become exposed to both unwanted human intrusion and white-nose syndrome, a pernicious disease that is decimating bats across America. As such, this species is now federally listed as an endangered species. As with most bats, disturbing them during hibernation can kill them. Stay out of caves.

WHITE-HAIRED GOLDENROD This lovely, showy flower is federally listed as a threatened species and can be found, sometimes in roped-off areas, in rock shelters and along cliffs. In fact, the white-haired goldenrod is native to the Red River Gorge and is found nowhere else in the world. Do not disturb this flower.

Hunting

According to the Daniel Boone National Forest website, Kentucky Department of Fish and Wildlife Resources regulations do, in fact, allow for both hunting and trapping in the Red River Gorge. Separate rules, regulations, and licenses govern the various hunting types and related seasons. Though no problems generally arise, hikers should take appropriate safety precautions for both themselves and their pets during hunting and trapping seasons.

Regulations

Rules and regulations differ a bit throughout the Red River Gorge area as detailed in this book, but in general they will follow both federal and Kentucky state-park regulations.

The federal rules and regulations, which cover the areas within the Red River Gorge Geological Area and the Clifty Wilderness, are as follows:

SANITATION

- Throw all garbage and litter in containers provided for this purpose or take it with you. Garbage containers, when provided, are reserved for visitors to the national forest, not for visitors or owners of private lands or lands under permit.

- Wash food and personal items away from drinking-water supplies. Use water faucets for drawing water only.

- Prevent pollution—keep garbage, litter, and foreign substances out of lakes, streams, and other water.

- Use toilets properly. Do not throw garbage, litter, fish cleanings, or other foreign substances in toilets and plumbing fixtures.

- To avoid creating potential sources of disease, dispose of sewer water (black water) only in sanitary dump stations.

- Collect kitchen and bath water (gray water) in a bucket or holding tank and empty in a dump station. Please do not use a drain hose for direct disposal.

- Wash personal items away from campground water faucets or pumps. Help keep the area clean for all to enjoy.

OPERATION OF VEHICLES

- Obey all traffic signs. State traffic laws apply to the national forests unless otherwise specified.

- When operating vehicles of any kind, do not damage the land or vegetation, or disturb wildlife. Avoid driving on unpaved wet roads or trails.

- Use cars, motorbikes, motorcycles, or other motor vehicles only for entering or leaving campgrounds and other recreation sites, unless areas or trails are specifically marked for them. Park only in marked parking areas.

- For the safety and convenience of others, please do not block, restrict, or interfere with the use of roads or trails.

- Operate bikes and other off-road vehicles to avoid damage to the forest. Obey area and trail restrictions on such use.

CAMPFIRES

- Obey restrictions on fires. Fires may be limited or prohibited at certain times of the year.

- Within campgrounds and other recreation sites, build fires only in fire rings, stoves, grills, or fireplaces provided for that purpose.

- Keep flammable materials away from campfires.

- You are responsible for keeping fires under control. Be sure your fire is completely extinguished before leaving.

- No camping or fire building is allowed within 100 feet of the base of any cliff or the back of any rock shelter.

- Campers and picnickers are encouraged to use charcoal or camp-stoves for cooking.

- If an open fire is necessary, dead and downed wood may be gathered. Do not cut living trees or standing dead trees.

- Never leave a fire unattended.

- Check for any fire-danger restrictions before starting a campfire.

CAMPING

- Use picnic sites, swimming beaches, and other day-use areas only between the hours of 6 a.m.–10 p.m.

- Campgrounds and other recreation sites can be used only for recreational purposes. Permanent use or use as a principal residence without authorization is not allowed.

- In campgrounds, camp only in those places specifically marked or provided.

- At least one person must occupy a camping area during the first night after camping equipment has been set up, unless permission has otherwise been granted by the forest ranger.

- Camping equipment cannot be left unattended for more than 24 hours without permission by the forest ranger.

- The federal government is not responsible for any loss or damage to personal property.

- Remove all personal property and trash when leaving.

FEE AREAS

- You must pay a fee to use certain developed sites and facilities. Such areas are clearly signed or posted as requiring a fee.

- Where fees are required, they must be paid before using the site, facility, equipment, or service furnished.

PROPERTY

- Do not carve, chop, cut, or damage any live trees.

- Preserve and protect your national forests. Leave natural areas the way you find them.

- Buildings, structures, or enclosed areas in national forests may be entered only when expressly opened to the public.

- Cultural sites, old cabins, and other structures, along with objects and artifacts associated with them, have historic or archeological value. Do not damage or remove any such historic or archaeological resources.

PUBLIC BEHAVIOR

- No fighting or boisterous behavior.

- Please keep noise at a reasonable level. Be courteous to your fellow visitors and observe quiet hours 10 p.m.–6 a.m. Keep music and voices low. Listen and enjoy the natural sounds.

- Do not operate generators after dark.

PETS AND ANIMALS

- Pets must always be restrained or kept on a leash.

- Pets are not allowed in swimming areas.

- Saddle, pack, or draft animals are allowed only in authorized areas.

- The most common nuisance in campgrounds is a loose dog. A usually obedient and innocent dog is often noisy when its owner is away. An unrestrained dog can harm campers, other pets, and wild animals.

- Always keep your pet on a leash in the campground, and never leave your dog unattended. On trails, dogs can interfere with people, horses, or bicycles. Keep your dog close to you and under control at all times.

- Pets are not allowed on the hiking trails or in the wooded areas of Natural Bridge State Resort Park.

BUSINESS ACTIVITIES

- Permits are required for 1) selling any merchandise; 2) posting or distributing any handbill, circular, paper, or notice; and 3) conducting or participating in a public meeting, assembly, or special event. Contact your district ranger office for more information.

AUDIO DEVICES

- Please operate any audio device, such as a radio or musical instrument, so that it will not disturb other forest visitors.

- A permit is required to operate a public-address system in or near a campsite or developed recreation site, or over a body of water.

FIREWORKS AND FIREARMS

- Use of fireworks or other explosives is prohibited within campgrounds and other recreation sites.

- Firing a gun is not allowed 1) in or within 150 yards of a residence, building, campsite, developed recreation site, or occupied area; 2) across or on a road or body of water; or 3) in any circumstance whereby any person may be injured or property damaged.

NATIONAL FOREST WILDERNESS

- Motor vehicles and motorized equipment are prohibited in designated wilderness areas.

- Preserve the wilderness. Leave only footprints; take only pictures.

GENERAL

- Be careful! Look out for natural hazards and dangers when you are in the forest.

- If you hike off trails or swim or dive in streams and lakes, you do so at your own risk. You are responsible for your own safety.

- Be especially alert for hazard trees—trees damaged by last year's storms that may fall across a trail, road, or recreation area.

Trail Etiquette

Always treat the trail, wildlife, and fellow hikers with respect. Here are some reminders.

- ★ Plan ahead in order to be self-sufficient at all times. That means carrying necessary supplies for changes in weather or other conditions. A well-planned trip brings satisfaction to you and to others.

- ★ Hike on open trails only.

- ★ In seasons or construction areas where road or trail closures may be a possibility, use the website addresses or phone numbers shown in the "Contacts" line for each of this guidebook's hikes to check conditions prior to heading out for your hike. And do not attempt to circumvent such closures.

- ★ Avoid trespassing on private land, and obtain all permits and authorization as required. Also, leave gates as you found them or as directed by signage.

★ Be courteous to other hikers, bikers, equestrians, and others you encounter on the trails.

★ Never spook wild animals or pets. An unannounced approach, a sudden movement, or a loud noise startles most critters, and a surprised animal can be dangerous to you, to others, and to itself. Give animals plenty of space.

★ Observe the yield signs around the region's trailheads and backcountry. Typically they advise hikers to yield to horses, and bikers to yield to both horses and hikers. By common courtesy on hills, hikers and bikers yield to any uphill traffic. When encountering mounted riders or horse packers, hikers can courteously step off the trail, on the downhill side if possible. So the horse can see and hear you, calmly greet the riders before they reach you and do not dart behind trees. Also resist the urge to pet horses unless you are invited to do so.

★ Stay on the existing trail and do not blaze any new trails.

★ Be sure to pack out what you pack in, leaving only your footprints. No one likes to see the trash someone else has left behind.

Tips on Enjoying Hiking in the Red River Gorge

The ruggedness of the Red River Gorge makes safety the number-one concern. Let someone know where you will be, where you plan to go within the area, and when you plan to return. Bring the proper gear—good boots, raingear, and all the safety essentials. In general, it is best to stay away from *climbing:* cliffs, arches, and rock shelters are all potentially dangerous. Unless you are an experienced rock climber with the proper gear, don't bother. You'll find views aplenty that will cost you little more than the exertion of hiking.

As for dogs, keep them on a leash. Better yet, don't bring them at all—unless you plan to clean up after them, it's best to leave them home. I have rarely seen people bring dogs on Red River Gorge trails.

Children are of special concern. I've included some very easy trails for very young children, even a few paved trails where strollers are easily pushed. But if you have children who are old enough to hike for shorter or even longer distances, it is imperative to warn them of the dangers inherent in cliffs. Most trails, including the paths over

Sky Bridge and Natural Bridge, are unfenced. I, for one, would not take my toddler to the Gorge—period.

Night hiking, though it is becoming increasingly popular in the United States, should be avoided here. Cliffs are far too sheer. To that advice I would add that certain camping areas are dubious. I've seen people camping on many ridgelines, including Auxier Ridge. With people wantonly breaking the rules, camping in dangerous areas and drinking, that seems a recipe for disaster. Use your common sense.

But none of this is in any way meant to discourage anyone from visiting and exploring the Gorge. Be safety-conscious and the danger is diminished dramatically. Stay on trails, be aware of your feet, and be especially aware of weather conditions. If you keep all this in mind, the Red River Gorge will be an experience to remember.

THIS 160-FOOT SUSPENSION BRIDGE SPANS THE RED RIVER.
(Hike 16, Sheltowee Trace–Bison Way Loop, page 105)

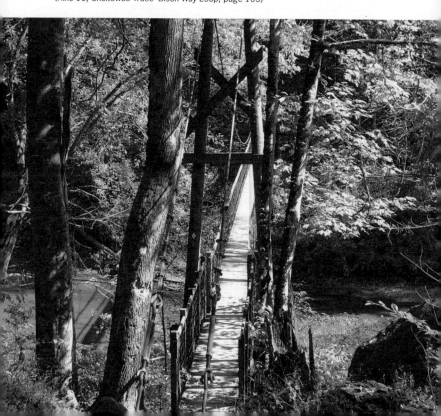

RED RIVER GORGE
GEOLOGICAL AREA

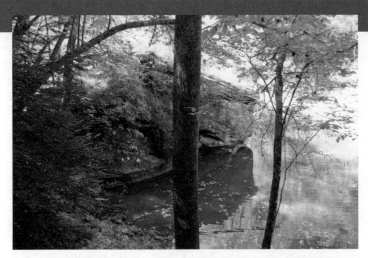

STOP AND TAKE IN THE BEAUTY OF THE RED RIVER FROM THIS SHADY SPOT.

1 ANGEL WINDOWS 32

2 CHIMNEY TOP ROCK, PRINCESS ARCH, AND HALF MOON ARCH 36

3 COURTHOUSE ROCK AND AUXIER RIDGE 41

4 D. BOON HUT 46

5 DOUBLE ARCH 50

6 GRAYS ARCH 55

7 KOOMER RIDGE AND HIDDEN ARCH 59

8 PINCH-EM-TIGHT RIDGE 64

9 ROCK BRIDGE ARCH 68

10 ROUGH TRAIL 73

11 SHELTOWEE TRACE 79

12 SILVERMINE ARCH AND CLIFF TRAIL 85

13 SKY BRIDGE 90

14 WHISTLING ARCH 94

15 WHITTLETON ARCH 98

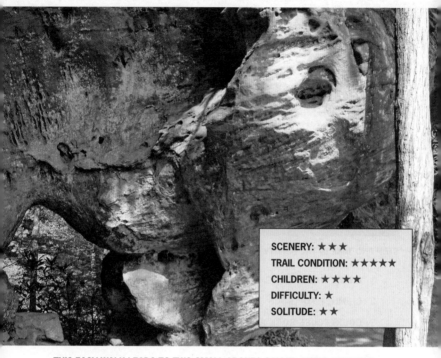

SCENERY: ★★★
TRAIL CONDITION: ★★★★★
CHILDREN: ★★★★
DIFFICULTY: ★
SOLITUDE: ★★

THIS EASY WALK LEADS TO TWO SMALL ARCHES CALLED ANGEL WINDOWS.

GPS TRAILHEAD COORDINATES: *Angel Windows Trailhead* N37° 47.932' W83° 35.473'

DISTANCE & CONFIGURATION: 0.5-mile out-and-back

HIGHLIGHTS: A wind-carved double arch and rock formations

HIKING TIME: 0.5 hour

ELEVATION: 1,110' at the trailhead, with no significant elevation gain or loss

ACCESS: Open 24/7; vehicle pass required for overnight parking

MAPS: USGS *Pomeroyton;* USFS *Red River Gorge Geological Area*

FACILITIES: None

WHEELCHAIR ACCESS: None

COMMENTS: Dangerous cliffs are present and should be avoided, especially by children.

CONTACTS: Daniel Boone National Forest, Cumberland Ranger District, Gladie Cultural-Environmental Learning Center: 606-663-8100, tinyurl.com/gladie

Overview

A short and easy hike, great for families, leads above the ravine of Parched Corn Creek to a double arch known as Angel Windows. Though the trail officially ends here, you can duck through one of the two windows, being extremely careful, especially with kids, and come out at the head of the ravine, with its stunning cliffs and rock shelters, seasonal waterfalls, and towering trees. A sign at the trailhead explains the strange name given the creek: Early explorers set up camps along the creek where they preserved their corn by dry roasting it. Settlers later logged the area, using the wood for their nearby farmsteads, as well as selling the wood. The forest seems to have recovered nicely. Be aware that no camping is allowed in the vicinity of Angel Windows. This is a great place to stop for lunch while exploring this area near the boundary of the Red River Gorge Geological Area and the Clifty Wilderness.

Route Details

From the parking lot, set out southwest on Angel Windows Trail 218. For a short distance the trail parallels the road, but it quickly enters a dense forest. The dirt trail descends very gradually, turning north and away from the road. A steep ravine will remain on the right side of the trail. On the left, a series of rock formations and outcrops accompanies the trail. After 0.25 mile, on a mostly steady grade, the trail passes a series of rock shelters to its terminus at Angel Windows. Though small, the two arches still provide vistas into a deep ravine just on the other side. Be careful at this trail's end; steep drop-offs flank either side of these "windows," which apparently were carved out by the wind.

The trail officially ends at the peculiar formation of Angel Windows, but you can explore the amphitheater-like grotto on the other side. Simply duck through the larger of the two arches, about 10 feet wide, and follow a well-beaten dirt path to the left along the impressive overhanging cliffs. At times, the sound of water will echo

Angel Windows

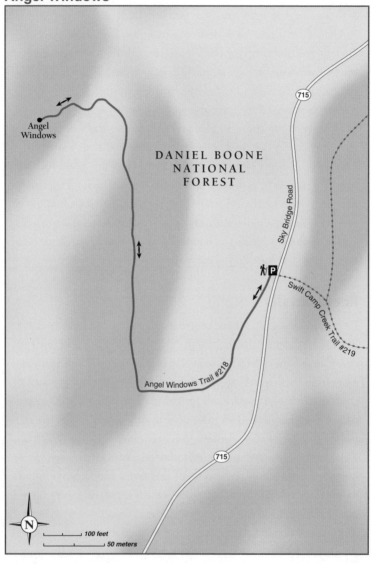

Angel
Windows

DANIEL BOONE
NATIONAL
FOREST

715

Sky Bridge Road

P

Swift Camp Creek Trail #219

Angel Windows Trail #218

715

N

100 feet
50 meters

through the ravine. The path follows the line of cliffs safely for about 100 yards. After that, it becomes rapidly dangerous. Be aware that wet rocks beyond this point can cause serious injury, so turn back where the path peters out.

Before you leave the head of this ravine, though, note how different the Angel Windows look from this side. At the right time of day, sunlight can be seen streaming through the windows. Notice, too, the sign on the tree that expressly forbids camping in this area. Head back on the path to the arches and return as you came. The trail gains mild elevation as it returns to the lot.

Directions

From Exit 40 off Bert T. Combs Mountain Parkway, go right on KY 15/KY 715 for 1 mile, and then follow KY 715 right for 4 miles to the Angel Windows Trailhead parking area, on the left. The trail begins at the southern edge of the lot.

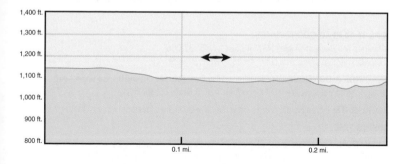

Chimney Top Rock, Princess Arch, and Half Moon Arch

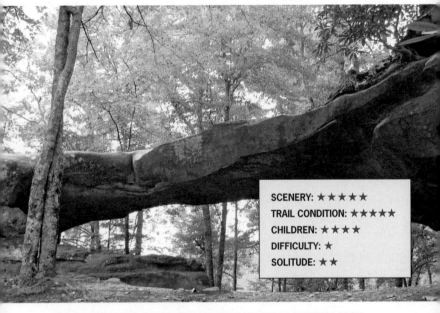

SCENERY: ★ ★ ★ ★
TRAIL CONDITION: ★ ★ ★ ★ ★
CHILDREN: ★ ★ ★ ★
DIFFICULTY: ★
SOLITUDE: ★ ★

THIS 32-FOOT-LONG SANDSTONE BRIDGE IS KNOWN AS PRINCESS ARCH.

GPS TRAILHEAD COORDINATES:
Chimney Top Recreation Area N37° 49.501' W83° 37.086'
Half Moon Arch parking area N37° 49.285' W83° 37.929'

DISTANCE & CONFIGURATION: Chimney Top Trail: 0.6-mile out-and-back; Princess Arch Trail: 0.7-mile out-and-back; Half Moon Arch Trail: 0.6-mile out-and-back

HIGHLIGHTS: Incredible panoramic views and two beautiful sandstone arches

HIKING TIME: 1 hour

ELEVATION: 1,207' feet at the Chimney Top Recreation Area parking lot, with no significant elevation gain or loss; 1,205' at the Half Moon pullout parking lot, with a loss of 190'

ACCESS: Open 24/7; vehicle pass required for overnight parking

MAPS: USGS *Pomeroyton*; USFS *Red River Gorge Geological Area*

FACILITIES: Restroom and picnic area at Chimney Top Recreation Area

WHEELCHAIR ACCESS: Yes, strollers and wheelchairs can be used on the paved trail to Chimney Top Rock.

COMMENTS: Dangerous cliffs are present and should be avoided, especially by children.

CONTACTS: Daniel Boone National Forest, Cumberland Ranger District, Gladie Cultural-Environmental Learning Center: 606-663-8100, tinyurl.com/gladie

Overview

The Chimney Top Recreation Area lies at the end of a dirt road at the far end of a steep ridge. Two short trails leave the parking lot and travel to sites not to be missed. The paved path to Chimney Top leads to an incredible lookout with a panoramic view over the Red River Gorge, the Chimney Top Creek Drainage, Half Moon Arch, Cloud Splitter Rock, and Pinch-Em-Tight Gap. At the opposite end of the parking lot, a regular dirt trail leads to Princess Arch, one of the prettiest of all the arches in the Red River Gorge area. This area has seen its share of deaths, more so than other parts of the Gorge, so be especially careful here. Trails are well kept and obvious; stay on them, keep children close, and enjoy the beautiful scenery. A third, unmarked hike leads to Half Moon Arch, a quick walk—though one that requires care—that is well worth the time. From Half Moon, you can look over the ravine and see Chimney Top Rock in a picture-perfect view.

Route Details

The trails to both Chimney Top Rock and Princess Arch start from the parking lot of Chimney Top Recreation Area, and both trailheads are clearly marked with signs. Start with the Chimney Top Rock Trail, which leaves the south end of the lot, at the far end of the roadway's loop, on a well-marked, paved trail. The next 0.3 mile passes through small pine trees, open enough to allow vistas to the south. A few benches along the way offer the chance to relax and take in the unsurpassed panoramas. The end of the trail is a promontory on the 200-foot-tall Chimney Top Rock. The stone walls and wood rails should be enough warning to keep away from the edges. Take in the sweeping vistas, among the best in the entire Red River Gorge Geological Area.

Chimney Top Rock, Princess Arch, and Half Moon Arch

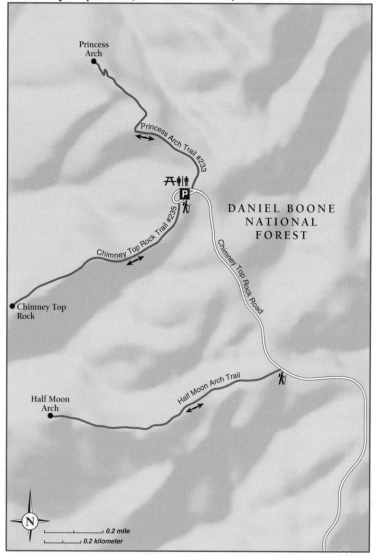

Now head back up the paved trail to the parking area and cross to the far end, past the outhouse, and north to the beginning of the roadway's loop. Watch for the sign indicating Princess Arch. This dirt trail is more rugged and natural. Princess Arch Trail follows a ridgetop through dry pinewoods 0.2 mile to the arch. It will appear as a long sandstone bridge, and the arch itself is not apparent, as it is directly below you. On the right, the plunge is a sheer drop-off into the forest.

From here, you can do a number of things. You can continue forward on the trail to another promontory on an unofficial trail. Note that some rock scrambling will be needed to get there, so children should probably be kept away. To find the promontory, continue over the bridge of Princess Arch, weaving left around a rock outcrop, descending a boulder, and continuing forward to the trail's terminus at a pinnacle rock with views over the Red River Gorge.

The second option, and probably the safer bet if you have children, is to get under the arch itself for a classic photo opportunity. To do this, turn around on the trail, as if heading back toward the lot, and watch for a user trail to the right. This trail descends a slightly steep rock that will prove treacherous if wet. At the bottom of this rock face, jog back to the right toward the arch, and you will plainly see the wide arch and the forest beyond it. Return as you came.

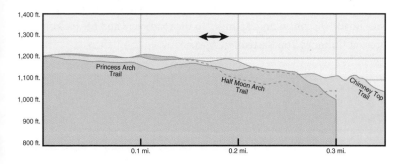

To see Half Moon Arch, return to your car and drive back down Chimney Top Rock Road about 0.3 mile. On the left side of the road, watch for a number of bear boxes and a small outhouse in the trees. Park in one of the pullouts on either side and follow an unmarked trail on the right (west) side of the road. This primitive trail climbs a very short distance and leads 0.3 mile along the ridge, passing numerous campsites. The path, wide and easily recognizable, drops after the campsites and narrows; in winter or during rain, this stretch of trail will likely resemble a creekbed. When the trail levels out on a sandstone ridge, where you can see Chimney Top Rock to the right, you will be close. At a flat, tabletop-like slab of sandstone, look to the left for a descent alongside the ridge. Go down carefully. Follow the cliff's edge and reach Half Moon Arch in only a few feet. The arch is big enough to slip through, but be aware of the cliff on the other side. Farther north along the ridge, the cliffs become towering, massive formations. Don't attempt to go any farther—these cliffs are sheer and the risk tremendous. Instead, enjoy the arch and return the way you came.

Directions

Take Exit 40 off Bert T. Combs Mountain Parkway. At the stop sign, go right on KY 15/KY 715 for 1 mile. Where the roads split in the small community of Pine Ridge, go right (north) on KY 715 for 2.2 miles and turn left onto gravel Chimney Top Rock Road (Forest Service Road 10), continuing 3.6 miles to the road's end and the parking area, at Chimney Top Recreation Area.

Courthouse Rock and Auxier Ridge

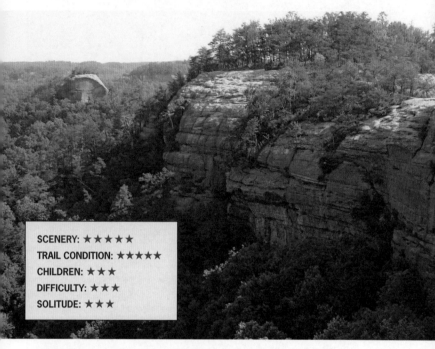

SCENERY: ★ ★ ★ ★ ★
TRAIL CONDITION: ★ ★ ★ ★ ★
CHILDREN: ★ ★ ★
DIFFICULTY: ★ ★ ★
SOLITUDE: ★ ★ ★

COURTHOUSE ROCK IS CLEARLY VISIBLE FROM THE AUXIER RIDGE TRAIL.

GPS TRAILHEAD COORDINATES: *Auxier Ridge Trailhead* N37° 49.212' W83° 40.856'

DISTANCE & CONFIGURATION: 5-mile balloon

HIKING TIME: 2.5 hours

HIGHLIGHTS: Rock formations, panoramic views, and wildflowers

ELEVATION: 1,355' at the trailhead, with a loss of 370'

ACCESS: Open 24/7; vehicle pass required for overnight parking

MAPS: USGS *Slade;* USFS *Red River Gorge Geological Area*

FACILITIES: Restroom

WHEELCHAIR ACCESS: None

COMMENTS: Dangerous cliffs are present and should be avoided, especially by children.

CONTACTS: Daniel Boone National Forest, Cumberland Ranger District, Gladie Cultural-Environmental Learning Center: 606-663-8100, tinyurl.com/gladie

Courthouse Rock and Auxier Ridge

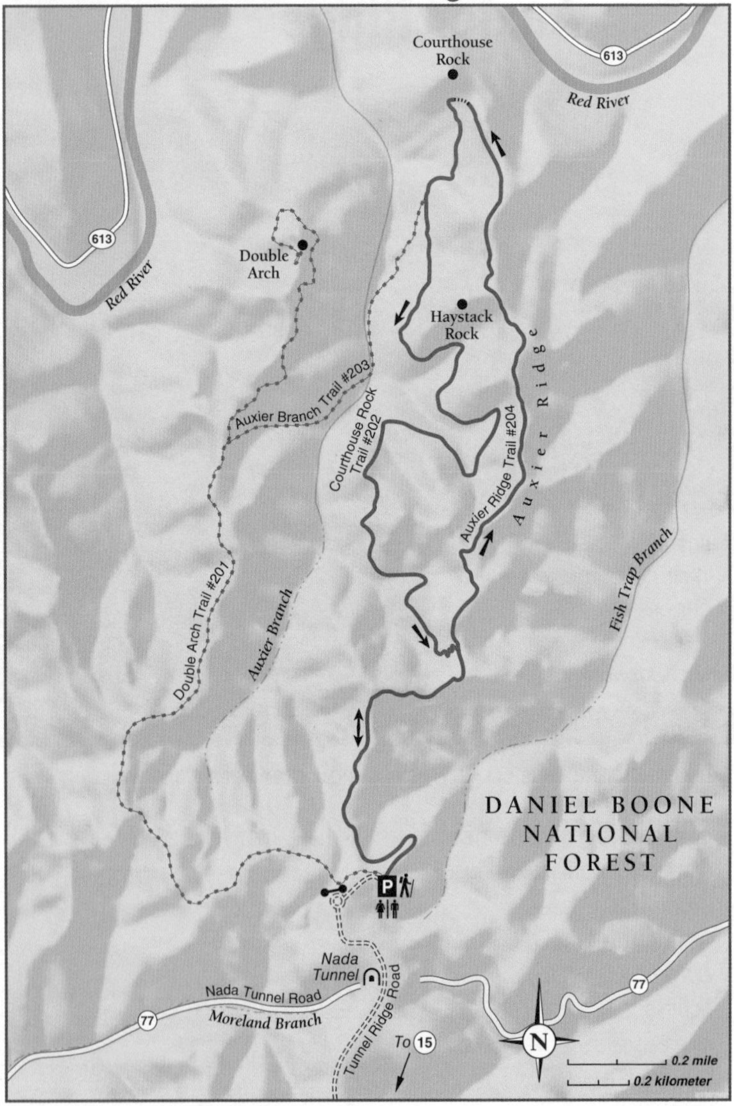

Courthouse
Rock

613

Red River

613

Double
Arch

Red River

Haystack
Rock

Auxier Branch Trail #203

Courthouse Rock
Trail #202

Auxier Ridge Trail #204

Auxier Ridge

Double Arch Trail #201

Auxier Branch

Fish Trap Branch

DANIEL BOONE
NATIONAL
FOREST

P

Nada
Tunnel

Nada Tunnel Road

77

Moreland Branch

Tunnel Ridge Road

To 15

77

N

0.2 mile

0.2 kilometer

Overview

The loop to Courthouse Rock offers the stunning clifftop views that make the Red River Gorge famous. From the highest points, you will see the Gorge itself, as well as vistas to Ravens Rock, Haystack Rock, and Double Arch. Half of the hike descends into the lush forest beneath some magnificent sandstone cliffs, and the second half follows Auxier Ridge through a recovering burn. Autumn colors make this hike even more spectacular, and spring is an excellent time to spot yellow and pink lady's slipper orchids.

Route Details

The Auxier Ridge Trail begins from the lot at the end of Tunnel Ridge Road. The first 500 feet of the trail descend quickly into the forest, and then the path levels out, traveling 0.8 mile north through lush rhododendron groves. The route climbs and falls gently, crossing forest damaged over time by pine beetles and fire. Soon the trail follows the length of Auxier Ridge. You will cross occasional sandstone outcrops and pass blooms of mountain laurels. At times the trail becomes mounds of eroded sand. At the 0.8-mile mark you'll reach the junction with Courthouse Rock Trail; this will be the return trail

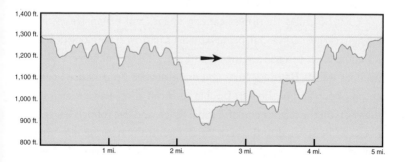

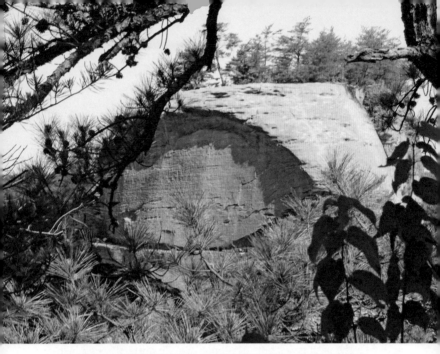

YOU WALK THROUGH A WOODED CANYON NEAR HIGH CLIFFS TO REACH COURTHOUSE ROCK.

for the loop. From here, you can go either clockwise or counterclockwise, depending on what you want to see first. If panoramic views are the first consideration, go right and stay on the Auxier Ridge Trail, headed north. The trail meanders along the fairly steady ridge with virtually no loss or gain of elevation. Here, the trail also briefly crosses the remnants of a fire that devastated the forest in 2010.

At 1.5 miles the forest canopy opens, and expansive vistas begin in earnest as the trail begins to skirt a narrow ridge along dizzying cliffs. First, you will see the magnificent cliffs of the Auxier Ridge itself, as well as Haystack Rock and dome-shaped Courthouse Rock, ahead of you and to the left. Double Arch can also easily be seen to the west, on the distant end of Tunnel Ridge, and flat-topped Ravens Rock can be spotted to the east. At one point the trail tightens and moves along precipitous drop-offs on either side; from here, the Red River Gorge carves an obvious gouge to the north. The pointed knob of Haystack Rock is on the left, and a large rock promontory looks over the forest into the cove between Tunnel Ridge and the Auxier

Ridge. At points, the trail narrows to bare rock no more than 30 feet across. Use caution.

Along the last forested stretch of the Auxier Ridge, the trail passes several illegal campsites. At 2.1 miles the trail reaches the base of towering Courthouse Rock. There is room for exploration around the rock itself, but you should in no way attempt to climb it. Instead, descend a steep staircase, newly built by the all-volunteer Red River Gorge Trail Crew, just to the east of Courthouse Rock and go south into the valley before you. At 2.4 miles you will reach the official end of the Auxier Ridge Trail at a junction. To the right is the Auxier Branch Trail, which leads to Double Arch; this can be made into a longer loop totaling 8.1 miles (see Hike 5, page 50). Instead, to complete this 5-mile loop hike, go left on Courthouse Rock Trail to return to the Auxier Ridge Trailhead.

Courthouse Rock Trail descends farther into a deep green, and surprisingly cool, forest. This is classic Red River Gorge low-elevation forest, and though glimpses of the overhanging cliffs are limited by the size of the trees, it makes for an easy and quiet walk. The trail crosses a series of small creeks that can become boggy in heavy rains. Hillsides of ferns, thickets of rhododendrons, and bigleaf magnolias (jungle-like in appearance) are common here. This section of trail meanders through the forest 2.1 miles, rounding the base of Haystack Rock along the way. As the trail nears its end, it climbs steadily back to the junction with the Auxier Ridge Trail at the 4.2-mile mark, where you will go right (south) 0.8 mile back to the lot.

Directions

From Exit 33 off Bert T. Combs Mountain Parkway, go 0.1 mile north on KY 11 and turn right on KY 15. In 3.5 miles go left onto gravel Tunnel Ridge Road (Forest Service Road 39). After 3 miles turn right into a parking lot at the Auxier Ridge Trailhead.

D. Boon Hut

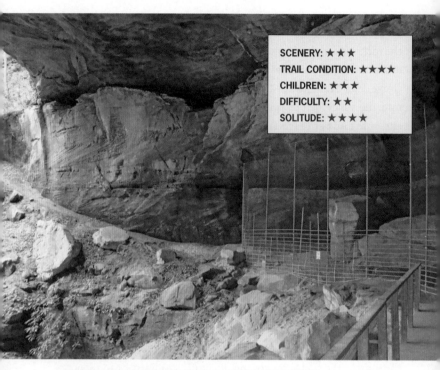

A FENCE PROTECTS THE HISTORICAL D. BOON ROCK CARVING.

GPS TRAILHEAD COORDINATES: *Grays Arch Picnic Area* N37° 48.481' W83° 39.456'

DISTANCE & CONFIGURATION: 1.5-mile loop

HIKING TIME: 1.5 hours

ELEVATION: 1,284' at the trailhead, with a loss of 395'

ACCESS: Open 24/7; vehicle pass required for overnight parking

MAPS: USGS *Slade;* USFS *Red River Gorge Geological Area*

FACILITIES: Restroom and picnic area

WHEELCHAIR ACCESS: None

COMMENTS: Overnight camping is prohibited at Grays Arch Picnic Area.

CONTACTS: Daniel Boone National Forest, Cumberland Ranger District, Gladie Cultural-Environmental Learning Center: 606-663-8100, tinyurl.com/gladie

Overview

Discovered in 1959 by three Kentuckians, a wooden hut with the name D. BOON carved on it was found in a remote rock shelter at the head of this rugged ravine. Speculation that the great Daniel Boone camped in this spot continues to this day. This now fenced-off shelter was also the site of a 19th-century niter mine; remains of wooden troughs and fireplaces are evidence that the site was used to produce potassium nitrate, a key ingredient of gunpowder. An easy 0.6-mile trail begins at the far end of Grays Arch Picnic Area and leads down a series of stairs to the rock overhang, making for a fairly easy out-and-back. But as long as you're going to visit the remains of the mysterious hut, why not make a more interesting loop of it? This roundabout route instead traverses down and along imposing cliffs on the Rough Trail, crossing a pleasant creek and ascending back to the spot of the historic hut before returning to the lot.

Route Details

From Grays Arch Picnic Area, start out on Grays Arch Trail. After 0.2 mile of mostly flat terrain, this dusty trail reaches a junction with the Rough Trail. Go left on the Rough Trail, descending dizzying sandstone slopes—be careful of wet rocks and keep an eye out for the white diamond blazes, which in some cases are printed on the rocks themselves, as the path is not always readily apparent. The views afforded here, however, are expansive, and you can easily see out over the valley you are descending into. Once the trail levels out, it then follows the base of stupendous and picturesque cliffs, descending to Martin's Fork at 0.75 mile and a sign pointing the way to the D. Boon Hut. Go left at this sign, heading gradually up to the head of the ravine. At 1.25 miles watch for another sign, which will point you to the right. To visit the hut, go upward and to the right at this sign toward the cliff walls, and follow the cliff to the right about 0.1 mile toward the long chain-link fence, site of the old hut and niter mine. Though for the most part you'll see virtually no trace of anything

D. Boon Hut

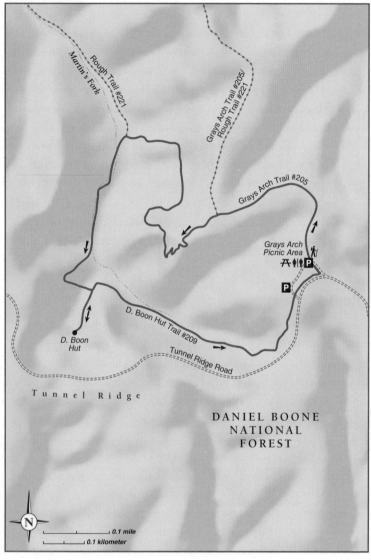

resembling a fully built hut, you will see evidence of human use. After reading the informative sign, return to the main D. Boon Hut Trail and continue in the direction you were going before the hut's spur trail, heading right and climbing up and out of the canyon to return to the western end of the Grays Arch parking area.

Directions

From Exit 33 off Bert T. Combs Mountain Parkway, go 0.1 mile north on KY 11 and turn right on KY 15. In 3.5 miles turn left onto gravel Tunnel Ridge Road (Forest Service Road 39). After 1 mile turn right into the parking lot for Grays Arch Picnic Area.

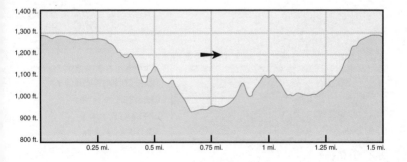

5 Double Arch

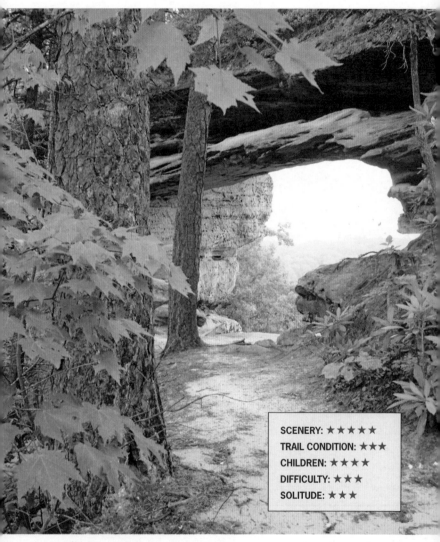

SCENERY: ★★★★★
TRAIL CONDITION: ★★★
CHILDREN: ★★★★
DIFFICULTY: ★★★
SOLITUDE: ★★★

A VISTA OF AUXIER RIDGE, HAYSTACK ROCK, AND COURTHOUSE ROCK AWAIT HIKERS AT DOUBLE ARCH.

GPS TRAILHEAD COORDINATES: *Auxier Ridge Trailhead* N37° 49.212' W83° 40.856'

DISTANCE & CONFIGURATION: 4.6-mile out-and-back

HIKING TIME: 2.5 hours

HIGHLIGHTS: Double Arch, towering cliffs, and rock formations

ELEVATION: 1,355' at the trailhead, with a loss of 247'

ACCESS: Open 24/7; vehicle pass required for overnight parking

MAPS: USGS *Slade;* USFS *Red River Gorge Geological Area*

FACILITIES: Restroom

WHEELCHAIR ACCESS: None

COMMENTS: Most of this trail follows an old U.S. Forest Service road open only to foot traffic. Dangerous cliffs are present and should be avoided, especially by children.

CONTACTS: Daniel Boone National Forest, Cumberland Ranger District, Gladie Cultural-Environmental Learning Center: 606-663-8100, tinyurl.com/gladie

Overview

Traversing a wooded ridge, the trail to Double Arch actually follows the old Tunnel Ridge Road, now closed to all but foot traffic. This makes for an easy, quick hike. The last stretch of trail begins from the end of the road at the old trailhead and promptly descends into a ravine, ambling in the shadow of substantial cliffs before rounding the end of the ridge and climbing to Double Arch, a two-tiered arch that offers not only shelter from the rain but also an unimpeded look across the densely forested cove to Auxier Ridge, Haystack Rock, and Courthouse Rock. This route makes for an easy out-and-back, though it can be combined with the Auxier Branch, Courthouse Rock, and Auxier Ridge Trails for a number of longer and more difficult loops.

Route Details

Beginning at the Auxier Ridge Trailhead parking lot, backtrack down the road about 300 feet to a turnaround and a locked gate marking the now-unused stretch of Tunnel Ridge Road. Though it wasn't always the case, this is the official beginning of the Double Arch Trail. The wide gravel road is pleasantly overhung by hardwood trees and features scenery both to the east and west, where cliffs and rock

Double Arch

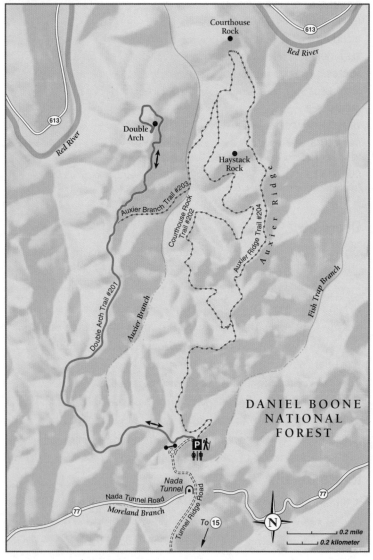

formations abound. The road continues for 1.4 miles, with gradual rises and falls, to the now-unused parking area on the right.

At the southern edge of the lot, two trails fan out into the forest. The unmarked trail to the right goes up the ridge to an overlook. Look for the trail sign indicating the Double Arch Trail, and instead go left and down a wooden stairway about 40 steps, descending quickly through a ravine into the shadow of these magnificent cliffs. Be careful during wet weather, as both the wooden stairway and rock along the trail can be slippery.

Now the trail evens out and becomes more level, but it is also more rugged, even primitive. In wet weather, this trail will likely turn extremely muddy. Also be prepared for the ankle-high poison ivy sprouting along the edge of the trail. But as rough as this trail can be, the payoff lies in the sheer cliffs that the trail follows beneath to the left. These sandstone cliffs are unsurpassed in their height and beauty. After 0.2 mile arrive at the junction with the Auxier Branch Trail, which you can use to form longer loops with the Courthouse Rock and Auxier Ridge Trails. If the arch is your primary destination, go left and stay on Double Arch Trail. Continue another 0.4 mile to a small, muddy stream coming down from the cliffs and look up and to the left to spot Double Arch in the orange cliffs about 100 feet above, the only notable double-span arch in the whole Red River Gorge area.

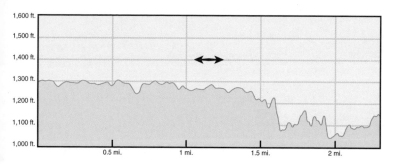

The last 0.3 mile continues through the dense forest, where the trail gradually circles the ridge and ascends to a final wooden staircase. At the top of the stairs, Double Arch is plainly visible immediately to the left. The upper arch is narrow and inaccessible, but the lower arch makes for a wide shelter, with plenty of boulders on which to sit. Looking east through the arch, you can easily see Haystack Rock and Auxier Ridge, and Courthouse Rock is far to the left. Use special caution here, as the cliffs beneath Double Arch are immediate and drastic. Just south of the arch and the stairway you will see steps carved into the sandstone wall, but it's probably best to avoid this. Likewise, beware of going too far along the edges beyond the arch.

After you've taken in the sights, return exactly as you came.

Directions

From Exit 33 off Bert T. Combs Mountain Parkway, go 0.1 mile north on KY 11 and turn right on KY 15. In 3.5 miles turn left onto gravel Tunnel Ridge Road (Forest Service Road 39). After 3 miles turn right into a parking lot at the Auxier Ridge Trailhead.

Grays Arch

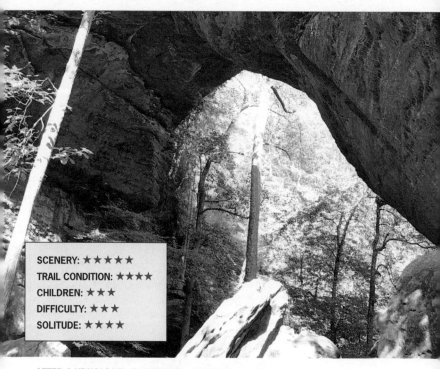

SCENERY: ★★★★★
TRAIL CONDITION: ★★★★
CHILDREN: ★★★
DIFFICULTY: ★★★
SOLITUDE: ★★★★

AFTER A HEAVY RAIN, A WATERFALL APPEARS AT GRAYS ARCH.

GPS TRAILHEAD COORDINATES: *Grays Arch Picnic Area* N37° 48.481' W83° 39.456'

DISTANCE & CONFIGURATION: 3.3-mile loop

HIKING TIME: 2 hours

ELEVATION: 1,284' at the trailhead, with a loss of 395'

ACCESS: Open 24/7; vehicle pass required for overnight parking

MAPS: USGS *Slade;* USFS *Red River Gorge Geological Area*

FACILITIES: Restroom and picnic area

WHEELCHAIR ACCESS: None

COMMENTS: Overnight camping is prohibited at Grays Arch Picnic Area.

CONTACTS: Daniel Boone National Forest, Cumberland Ranger District, Gladie Cultural-Environmental Learning Center: 606-663-8100, tinyurl.com/gladie

Grays Arch

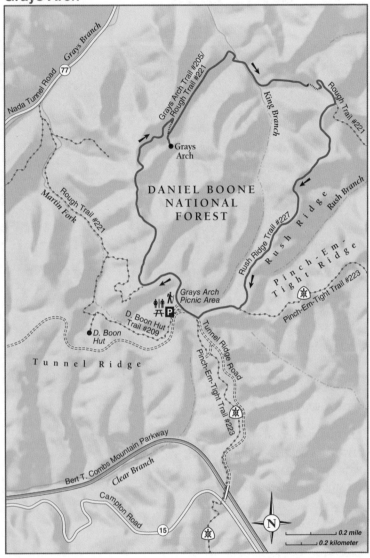

Overview

One of the quickest and easiest ways to see one of the most famous arches in the Red River Gorge region is to make a short ramble through the forest to Grays Arch. Perched above an impressive over-hang of cliffs dripping a steady pulse of water into a huge amphi-theater of sandstone, Grays Arch spans 80 feet and stands 50 feet. It is reportedly the biggest arch in the entire Red River Gorge area. Because of its popularity, the 2.2-mile round-trip trail can become congested with families and large groups on summer weekends, but it's worth a visit nevertheless. It's tempting to follow suit and make this an out-and-back trip, but for a taste of solitude and the varying topography of the area, add an extra mile and make this a stunning loop through deep forests and over cool creeks.

Route Details

From Grays Arch Picnic Area, begin on Grays Arch Trail, hiking under towering oaks and pines. After 0.2 mile turn right on the Rough Trail, one of the longer trails in the area. In another 0.2 mile, the trail crosses an open meadow and then begins to descend into the ravine. Watch for the arch to your right. Go another 0.5 mile and walk down the steep staircases to what appears to be a junction; the Rough

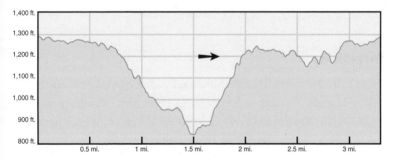

Trail continues, turning sharply left at a clear sign posted close to the ground. Instead go right down the trail to the amphitheater of striated sandstone. In the past, a number of poor user trails ascended to the arch, and as a result people trampled the ground of this rock shelter, which is home to numerous ferns and other plants. Do not cross the fence that has since been erected; the land here is recovering. Follow the newly built trail up and to the left to the underside of the arch.

For many people, a trip to Grays Arch is enough, and most visitors typically return the way they came, making a 2.2-mile out-and-back trip. But you can also make a 3.3-mile loop by continuing on the Rough Trail. After visiting the arch, go back to the Rough Trail. Instead of going left, which returns to the picnic area, go right to continue on the Rough Trail. In 0.2 mile the trail descends to King Branch, which flows through a forested flat and is worth the hike just to feel the coolness of the air. After crossing the creek three times on small footbridges and climbing a series of steps out of the hollow, continue up the ridge to the Rush Ridge Trail. By now, you've traveled 2 miles. Turn right onto the Rush Ridge Trail, which follows a level path for 1 mile over this ridge, much of which was burned in 2010. The forest is recovering, and views open out to Pinch-Em-Tight Ridge. At the end of Rush Ridge Trail, turn right on Pinch-Em-Tight Trail, part of the Sheltowee Trace, and go 0.2 mile to Tunnel Ridge Road. Return to your car by a short 0.1-mile walk to the right, following the road back to Grays Arch Picnic Area.

Directions

From Exit 33 off Bert T. Combs Mountain Parkway, go 0.1 mile north on KY 11 and turn right on KY 15. In 3.5 miles turn left onto gravel Tunnel Ridge Road (Forest Service Road 39). After 1 mile turn right into a parking lot for Grays Arch Picnic Area.

7 Koomer Ridge and Hidden Arch

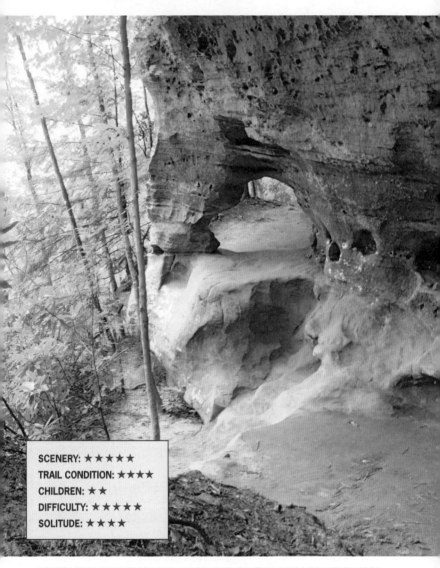

SCENERY: ★ ★ ★ ★ ★
TRAIL CONDITION: ★ ★ ★ ★
CHILDREN: ★ ★
DIFFICULTY: ★ ★ ★ ★ ★
SOLITUDE: ★ ★ ★ ★

DESPITE THE LANDMARK'S NAME, A WELL-MARKED TRAIL LEADS TO HIDDEN ARCH.

Koomer Ridge and Hidden Arch

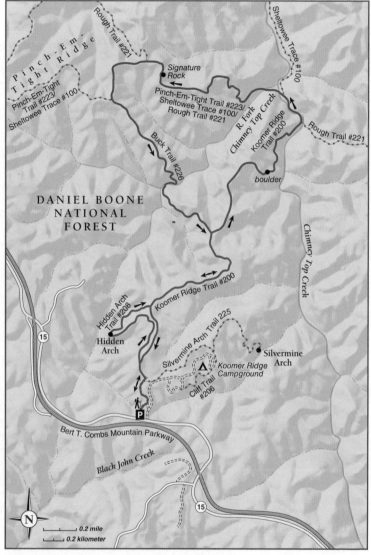

GPS TRAILHEAD COORDINATES: *Koomer Ridge Trailhead* N37° 46.888' W83° 38.164'

DISTANCE & CONFIGURATION: 7.9-mile double loop

HIKING TIME: 5.5 hours

HIGHLIGHTS: Hidden Arch, two forks of Chimney Top Creek, ridgeline views, cliffs, and rock formations

ELEVATION: 1,245' at the trailhead, descending to 736'

ACCESS: Open 24/7; vehicle pass required for overnight parking

MAPS: USGS *Slade;* USFS *Red River Gorge Geological Area*

FACILITIES: Restrooms and water available at campground

WHEELCHAIR ACCESS: None

COMMENTS: Dangerous cliffs are present and should be avoided, especially by children.

CONTACTS: Daniel Boone National Forest, Cumberland Ranger District, Gladie Cultural-Environmental Learning Center: 606-663-8100, tinyurl.com/gladie

Overview

To the north of Koomer Ridge Campground lies some of the most amazing terrain in the Red River Gorge area. Around Koomer Ridge, a double loop surveys the best of the region. You will enjoy Hidden Arch, rock shelters, and a deep woodsy walk along several forks of Chimney Top Creek. Spanning more than 600 feet of elevation, the trail climbs and descends with towering views over the surrounding ravines. This hike requires several stream crossings, which are not at all difficult when the water runs low. Give yourself plenty of time

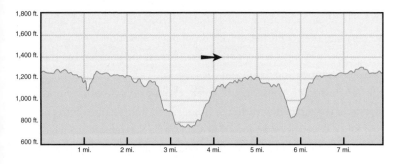

for this hike. Flowing creeks sparkling beneath cliffs and coursing around house-size boulders, coupled with breathtaking vistas of the sometimes cloud-draped valleys, enchant you to stop and contemplate the beauty of the Red River Gorge country.

Route Details

The trailhead for Koomer Ridge and Hidden Arch is an easy 500 feet from the parking lot, adjacent to the campground host's site. Follow this combination trail for Koomer Ridge, Hidden Arch, and Silvermine Arch for 0.2 mile through the campground to a junction, and then go left and to the north, following signs for the Hidden Arch Trail. Cross the road and pass a vault toilet among several campsites, continuing away from the campground and onto the trail. At 0.3 mile the trail splits. Go left and bear northwest here, following Hidden Arch Trail to impressive overhanging sandstone cliffs and Hidden Arch, so named because if you come from the opposite direction, you may well miss it.

Continuing on Hidden Arch Trail, connect with the Koomer Ridge Trail at 1 mile. Go left and roughly northeast on the Koomer Ridge Trail, following a sign for the Rough Trail. Now the path follows what is, in heavy rains, a quite boggy area, making it perfect for spotting lady's slipper orchids and irises March–May. In 0.5 mile the trail passes the junction with the Buck Trail, which will end one of the loops; for now, continue straight on Koomer Ridge Trail another 0.3 mile to a large illegal campsite at the edge of the ridge. Stop for the breathtaking scenery and then continue, quickly dropping in elevation.

After passing a large, pockmarked limestone boulder, the trail reaches Chimney Top Creek and the junction with the Rough Trail at the 3.1-mile mark. This languid creek, choked occasionally by massive boulders draped with ferns, flows north and empties into the Red River. On either side, towering cliffs cradle this remote stretch of forest, where you can certainly find some solitude.

Go left on the Rough Trail, continuing to a creek crossing and heading downstream 0.3 mile to a junction with the Sheltowee Trace. Turn left (west) here on the combination Rough Trail and Sheltowee

Trace, crossing the creek and heading into a lush forest. Follow the Right Fork of Chimney Top Creek upstream a short distance before climbing steadily through the remnants of a 1999 fire. Look on the ground, where white agates litter the exposed sandstone. The trail crosses Signature Rock, a smooth stone outcrop with imposing views over the burn to the ridges in the distance. Continuing upward, the trail intersects Pinch-Em-Tight Trail at 4.5 miles. Here, go left on the combined Pinch-Em-Tight and Sheltowee Trace for 0.4 mile to the Buck Trail.

Turn left and roughly southeast on the Buck Trail, an easy 1.5-mile jaunt that leads back to the Koomer Ridge Trail. You will descend to and ford the Right Fork of Chimney Top Creek at the 5.8-mile mark before climbing back to the junction with Koomer Ridge Trail. From this final junction, stay on Koomer Ridge Trail for 1.3 miles to return to the campground and complete the loop.

Directions

From Exit 33 off Bert T. Combs Mountain Parkway, go 0.1 mile north on KY 11 and turn right on KY 15. In 5.1 miles turn left at the sign for Koomer Ridge Campground and immediately turn left onto a short spur road to the trailhead parking area.

8 Pinch-Em-Tight Ridge

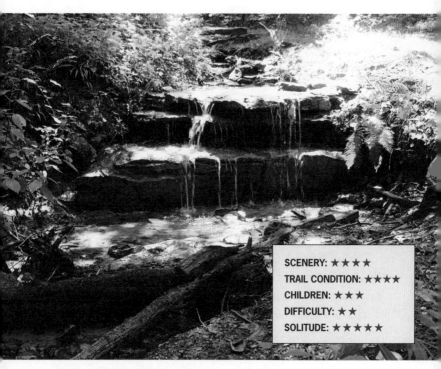

CHECK OUT RUSH BRANCH WATERFALL ALONG THE ROUGH TRAIL.

GPS TRAILHEAD COORDINATES: *Grays Arch Picnic Area* N37° 48.481' W83° 39.456'

DISTANCE & CONFIGURATION: 3.8-mile loop

HIKING TIME: 2.5 hours

ELEVATION: 1,267' at the trailhead, with a loss of 427'

ACCESS: Open 24/7; vehicle pass required for overnight parking

MAPS: USGS *Slade;* USFS *Red River Gorge Geological Area*

FACILITIES: Restroom and picnic area

WHEELCHAIR ACCESS: None

COMMENTS: Overnight camping is prohibited at Grays Arch Picnic Area.

CONTACTS: Daniel Boone National Forest, Cumberland Ranger District, Gladie Cultural-Environmental Learning Center: 606-663-8100, tinyurl.com/gladie

Overview

In 2010 a fire roared through this area, burning a great deal of the forest along Rush Ridge, though Pinch-Em-Tight Ridge was spared. This loop follows both ridges, providing chances to see both the open high-elevation forest along the Pinch-Em-Tight Trail and the recovering burn on Rush Ridge, whose fire-opened canopies allow views over the surrounding ridges and ravines. In between the two ridges, the Rough Trail dives to a series of lovely creeks in a deep, green basin. This loop is sure to be quiet and nearly hiker-free, making it a great place to relax in the peaceful forest. Especially wonderful are the little waterfalls on Rush Branch.

Route Details

If you parked at Grays Arch Picnic Area, go back to Tunnel Ridge Road and walk a short distance south. Watch on the east side of the road for the trailhead sign. From Tunnel Ridge Road, head east on Pinch-Em-Tight Trail, which for this section is part of the Sheltowee Trace—you'll see the white turtle blazes on trees along the way. In 0.2 mile stay to the right at the intersection with the Rush Ridge Trail, which will be the return route. This section of trail moves steadily on level ground through a dry forest of towering pines and hardwoods, with occasional views out to distant ridges and over the deep hollows. At 1.3 miles the Buck Trail intersects on the right (and heads 1 mile to the Koomer Ridge Trail, opening up more possibilities for longer loops and backpacking adventures); to continue this hike, go left at the junction, following signs toward the Rough Trail.

From here, Pinch-Em-Tight Trail descends 0.4 mile to the Rough Trail. Go left on the Rough Trail toward Grays Arch. The path immediately begins its nearly 400-foot descent into a lush gorge of rhododendrons to the cascading Rush Branch, where the air, even in summer, can be markedly cooler. Cross this creek and another small stream on two small log bridges and immediately begin the steep climb to the Rush Ridge Trailhead at 2.6 miles. Go left on the Rush

Pinch-Em-Tight Ridge

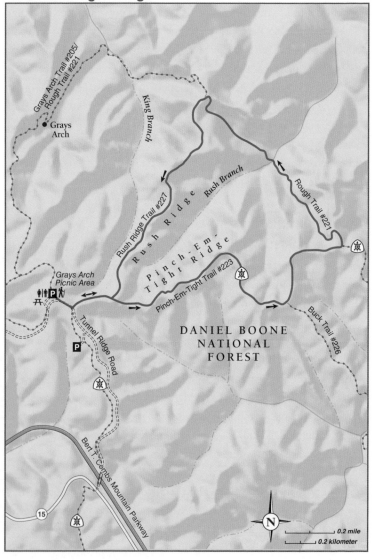

Ridge Trail through the remains of the 2010 burn for 1 mile, returning to the junction with Pinch-Em-Tight Trail. From there, go right to cover the remaining 0.2 mile to Tunnel Ridge Road. Of course, this loop can also be reversed, or even expanded to connect with either the Koomer Ridge trail system or the Grays Arch area.

Directions

From Exit 33 off Bert T. Combs Mountain Parkway, go 0.1 mile north on KY 11 and turn right on KY 15. In 3.5 miles turn left onto gravel Tunnel Ridge Road (Forest Service Road 39). After 1 mile turn right into the parking lot for Grays Arch Picnic Area.

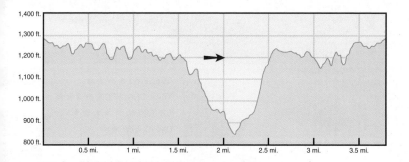

9 Rock Bridge Arch

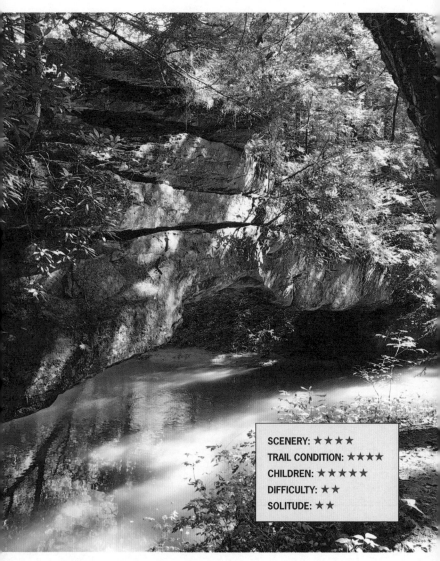

SCENERY: ★★★★
TRAIL CONDITION: ★★★★
CHILDREN: ★★★★★
DIFFICULTY: ★★
SOLITUDE: ★★

ROCK BRIDGE ARCH FORMS A NATURAL BRIDGE OVER SWIFT CAMP CREEK.

GPS TRAILHEAD COORDINATES: *Rock Bridge Recreation Area*
N37° 46.208' W83° 34.008'

DISTANCE & CONFIGURATION: 1.4-mile loop

HIKING TIME: 1 hour

HIGHLIGHTS: Rock Bridge Arch, old-growth forest, numerous creeks, and a waterfall

ELEVATION: 1,144' at the trailhead, descending to 887'

ACCESS: Open 24/7; vehicle pass required for overnight parking

MAPS: USGS *Pomeroyton;* USFS *Red River Gorge Geological Area*

FACILITIES: Restrooms and picnic area

WHEELCHAIR ACCESS: None

COMMENTS: Camping is prohibited at Rock Bridge Recreation Area.

CONTACTS: Daniel Boone National Forest, Cumberland Ranger District, Gladie Cultural-Environmental Learning Center: 606-663-8100, tinyurl.com/gladie

Overview

This easy path, great for kids, visits some of the biggest trees in the area, including eastern hemlocks, which give parts of this trail a vaulted feel. Tangles of flowering rhododendrons, mountain laurels, and holly bushes line the trail. The path follows Rock Bridge Fork and Swift Camp Creek, passing a waterfall and Rock Bridge Arch, the only rock bridge in the Red River Gorge area that lives up to its name, as it actually spans running water. This is what is known as a waterfall arch, where a waterfall once cut through the less-resistant rock, leaving this quiet span. Stop at an overlook on the return path.

Route Details

Starting from the picnic area in the Rock Bridge Recreation Area, look for the big painted signpost detailing Rock Bridge Arch's formation. Note that Rock Bridge Trail was paved a number of years ago, so it is broken up in places and generally uneven; it's easy enough for foot travel but not accessible for wheelchairs and strollers.

The trail drops in elevation quickly, descending a number of steps (and losing 150 feet of elevation) into a particularly lush forest of old-growth hemlocks, holly, rhododendrons, mountain laurels,

Rock Bridge Arch

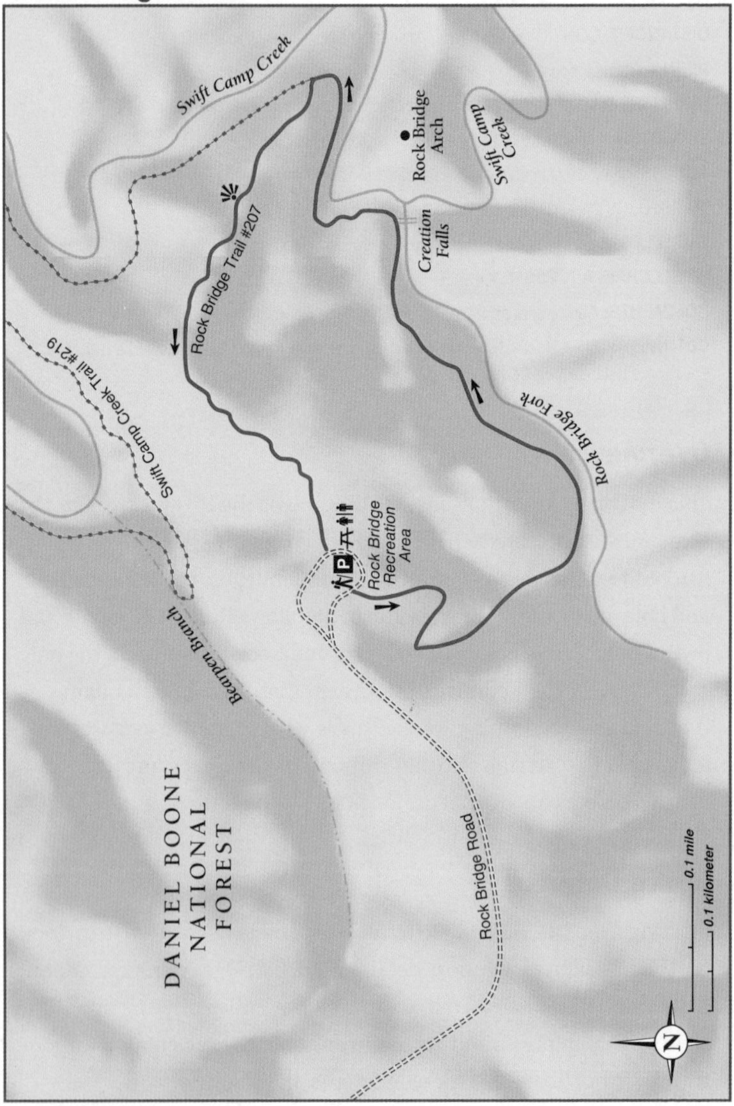

Swift Camp Creek

Rock Bridge Arch

Swift Camp Creek

Creation Falls

Rock Bridge Trail #207

Swift Camp Creek Trail #219

Rock Bridge Fork

Rock Bridge Recreation Area

Bearpen Branch

DANIEL BOONE NATIONAL FOREST

Rock Bridge Road

0.1 mile
0.1 kilometer

and ferns. The trail passes two rock shelters, descending even more steps to where it follows a small seasonal stream about 0.25 mile to a truly magnificent forest. The trees begin to tower, producing a cathedral-like effect in the darkened understory. About 0.3 mile farther, the small tributary the trail has been following joins Rock Bridge Fork, and at 0.5 mile the hike arrives at Creation Falls on the fork. There is plenty of room to explore around Creation Falls, and the creek above the falls is easy to cross. Do not, however, get close to the falls themselves, as the rock will likely be very slippery and the drop-off is enough to cause an injury. It's best to stay along the sandy beaches that line the creek.

Just downstream from the falls, Rock Bridge Fork quickly joins the far-larger Swift Camp Creek. Continue on the trail a short distance, past an overlook of Creation Falls and the confluence of Rock Bridge Fork with Swift Camp Creek, to Rock Bridge Arch at 0.6 mile. Rock Bridge Arch is a bit different in that it is actually composed of limestone rather than the more dominant sandstone arches of the Red River Gorge. Climbing the arch is not easy and requires a bit of scrambling. Again, please use caution.

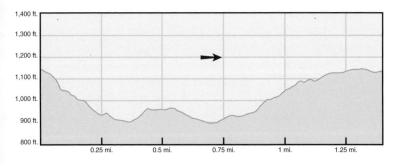

At the arch itself, there is a confusing junction; ignore the trail to the left and go to the right over a small footbridge to continue past the arch and to finish the loop. At 0.9 mile Rock Bridge Trail meets Swift Camp Creek Trail, which continues along the creek deep into the Clifty Wilderness. Follow Rock Bridge Trail and continue uphill, stopping at a stone-walled overlook and a bench, to return to the picnic area. The trail emerges near some pit toilets, across the picnic area from the original trailhead.

Directions

Take Exit 40 off Bert T. Combs Mountain Parkway. At the stop sign, turn right on KY 15/KY 715 for 1 mile. Where the roads split in the small community of Pine Ridge, go right (north) 1 mile on KY 715, and then turn right onto gravel Rock Bridge Road (Forest Service Road 24). Continue 3 miles to the road's end and the parking area at Rock Bridge Recreation Area.

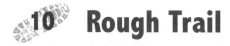

10 Rough Trail

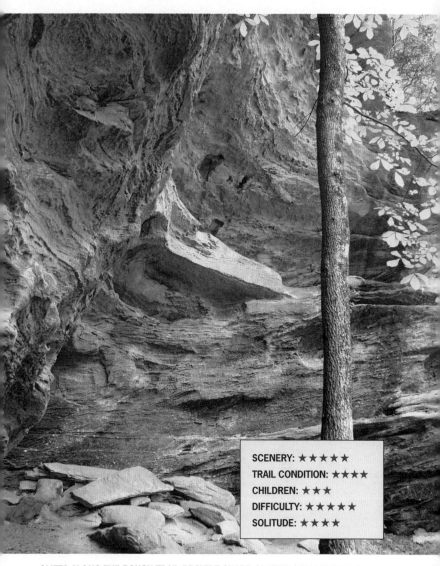

SCENERY: ★★★★★
TRAIL CONDITION: ★★★★
CHILDREN: ★★★
DIFFICULTY: ★★★★★
SOLITUDE: ★★★★

CLIFFS ALONG THE ROUGH TRAIL PROVIDE SHADE ON THIS CHALLENGING PATH.

The Rough Trail

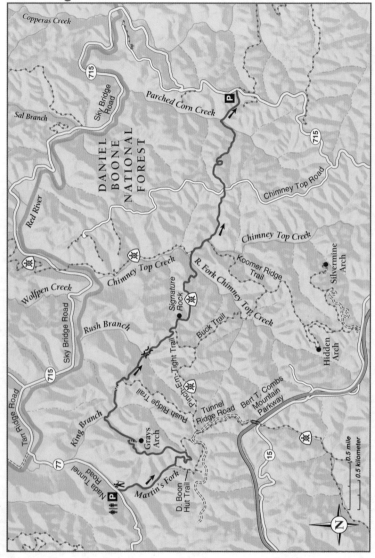

GPS TRAILHEAD COORDINATES: *Martin's Fork Trailhead* N37° 49.159' W83° 40.051'
Rough Trail and Swift Camp Creek Trailhead N37° 48.110' W83° 35.451'

DISTANCE & CONFIGURATION: 7.7-mile point-to-point

HIGHLIGHTS: Rugged but scenic forest, ridgetop and creekside hikes, Grays Arch, and backpacking opportunities

HIKING TIME: 8 hours

ELEVATION: 784' at the trailhead, ascending to 1,267'

ACCESS: Open 24/7; vehicle pass required for overnight parking

MAPS: USGS *Slade* and *Pomeroyton;* USFS *Red River Gorge Geological Area*

FACILITIES: Restrooms at Martin's Fork Trailhead

WHEELCHAIR ACCESS: None

COMMENTS: This is a long and difficult trail, best done as a shuttle or as an extended backpacking trip. Dangerous cliffs are present and should be avoided, especially by children.

CONTACTS: Daniel Boone National Forest, Cumberland Ranger District, Gladie Cultural-Environmental Learning Center: 606-663-8100, tinyurl.com/gladie

Overview

The Rough Trail, without a doubt, lives up to its name. That said, it is also likely the single-best long trail in the whole of the Red River Gorge. To do the entire trail demands endurance, as the path climbs no fewer than five ridges. Still, it can be done in a single day, or it can be tackled as a backpacking adventure. Along the way, there are

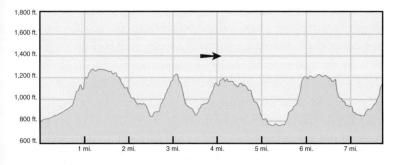

plenty of creeks and amazing rock formations, including iconic Grays Arch. The forest constantly changes with the elevation, so this trail serves as a lesson in the ecosystem of the Red River Gorge, both the shadier, greener mixed mesophytic forest and the drier, higher elevation stands where pines and oaks predominate.

Route Details

The best place to start the trail is at the far-busier Martin's Fork Trailhead, which is used by rock climbers as well as day hikers and backpackers. By starting early, you'll avoid not only the crowds at the beginning of the trail, which include the numerous visitors to Grays Arch, but you'll also maintain your solitude as you progress into the quieter, less-traveled sections of the trail.

From the Martin's Fork Trailhead, cross the road to the obvious sign. From here, the first 0.7 mile of the Rough Trail follows the lowland bottoms of Martin's Fork, crossing and recrossing several footbridges along the way. This section is lovely and densely green; however, it is also marred by the number of old campsites that the U.S. Forest Service has closed for rehabilitation, resulting in a damaged look. Along this section, two spur trails, Military Wall and Left Flank Trails, veer off on either side to rock-climbing areas.

At a small creek, the Rough Trail intersects the D. Boon Hut Trail, which climbs a gully to the right. Continue straight on the Rough Trail into one of the best parts of this hike. You quickly climb more than 350 feet through an array of dazzling cliffs over the course of 0.4 mile; then the trail climbs a somewhat confusing sandstone slope—watch for blazes and footsteps in the sand. At the top of the ridge, outlooks abound over the ravines of Martin's Fork. In another 0.1 mile, the trail reaches Grays Arch Trail.

At this intersection, go left to stay on the Rough Trail. This section sees a lot of business at almost any time of year, and it is wide enough and trampled enough to prove it. The path sets out into a high-elevation forest of tall oaks, crosses a wide and weedy meadow, and then descends into the forest. At a railing on the right side of the trail, particularly when the leaves have fallen, the first glimpse of Grays Arch is visible. After 0.8 mile past the Grays Arch junction, the Rough Trail descends two long stairways to a junction, with a sign pointing left for the Rough Trail. At this point, the trail has descended 270 feet from the top of the ridge. Look up before you, and Grays Arch is clearly visible. The spur trail to the right leads to an impressive rock overhang and an excellent view of the arch.

From this junction, the trail continues 1.1 miles deeper into the forest, heading down another 170 feet to a beautiful stream crossing at King Branch in a forested bottom, and then begins another steep ascent, climbing 400 feet to a junction with the Rush Ridge Trail. Go left to continue on the Rough Trail.

The next 1.2 miles lead to the Pinch-Em-Tight Trail, descending and reascending nearly 400 feet, and it is in this section where navigating may lead to some confusion. The trail, not entirely clearly marked at this point, descends some slickrock into a gully hemmed in by rock shelters; watch for blazes and signs, and follow the contours of the gully to the left—part of a seasonal creekbed that can make this even more unnerving. At the intersection with Pinch-Em-Tight Trail, continue to the left on the combination Rough Trail/Sheltowee Trace—from here, you'll see both white diamond and turtle blazes.

The next 1.3-mile section follows the ridge, crossing an overlook at Signature Rock, and then descends a steep and sometimes washed-out trail to the first of several crossings in the Chimney Top Creek drainage. This part of the hike skirts along the edge of the burn, which opens views over the rugged country to the north. Note that during the height of summer, this section of trail can be extremely hot.

After fording the Right Fork of Chimney Top Creek, followed by the larger Chimney Top Creek, the Sheltowee Trace veers left. Follow the Rough Trail to the right.

From here, cross Chimney Top Creek two more times in 0.2 mile on a mostly level bottomland in the heart of the drainage, the last crossing at a junction with Koomer Ridge Trail. The Rough Trail heads over the creek to the left and immediately begins climbing a rough stretch of terrain, which includes large downed trees and mud. In less than 0.7 mile the trail gains 450 feet to reach a parking area on Chimney Top Road, leveling out about halfway up the ridge.

For some, this may be journey enough. The trailhead on Chimney Top Road can mark a good place to shuttle as well, but it's worth it to continue the final 2 miles through what is probably the quietest section of the Rough Trail. Continue past the lot and into the woods, crossing the dirt road, and then follow a ridge into a stand of large deciduous trees. The trail descends into the ravine of Parched Corn Creek, passing stellar rock shelters and cliffs along the way. When the trail reaches the creek, it follows it for a distance, crosses it on a footbridge, and then begins a modest climb to the parking area on KY 715 that marks the official end of the Rough Trail and the beginning of the Swift Camp Creek Trailhead.

Directions

For the Martin's Fork Trailhead, take Exit 33 off Bert T. Combs Mountain Parkway and go north on KY 11 to the junction of KY 15. Go left on KY 15 for 1.5 miles to KY 77. Go right on KY 77 and travel 3.3 miles (the road goes through Nada Tunnel) to the trailhead parking on the left.

For the Rough Trail and Swift Camp Creek Trailhead, take Exit 40 off Bert T. Combs Mountain Parkway, go right on KY 15/715 for 1 mile, and then follow KY 715 right for 4.2 miles to the parking area, on the left.

Sheltowee Trace

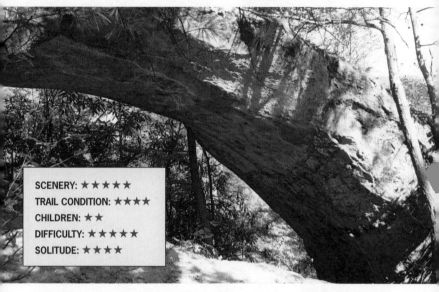

SCENERY: ★ ★ ★ ★ ★
TRAIL CONDITION: ★ ★ ★ ★
CHILDREN: ★ ★
DIFFICULTY: ★ ★ ★ ★ ★
SOLITUDE: ★ ★ ★ ★

A DIFFICULT TRAIL MEANS YOU'LL LIKELY FIND SOLITUDE AT INDIAN ARCH.

GPS TRAILHEAD COORDINATES: *Corner Ridge Trailhead* N37° 53.186' W83° 35.600'
Pinch-Em-Tight Trailhead N37° 48.321' W83° 39.315'

DISTANCE & CONFIGURATION: 14-mile point-to-point

HIGHLIGHTS: A sandstone arch, cliff formations, rugged forest trails, creekside hiking, excellent backpacking opportunities, and a swinging bridge over the Red River

HIKING TIME: 11 hours

ELEVATION: 1,283' at the trailhead, descending to 705'

ACCESS: Open 24/7; vehicle pass required for overnight parking

MAPS: USGS *Pomeroyton* and *Slade;* USFS *Red River Gorge Geological Area*

FACILITIES: None

WHEELCHAIR ACCESS: None

COMMENTS: This trail is best done as a shuttle. Leave one vehicle at Corner Ridge Trailhead, the beginning point, and the second at Pinch-Em-Tight Trailhead on Tunnel Ridge Road. Dangerous cliffs are present and should be avoided, especially by children.

CONTACTS: Daniel Boone National Forest, Cumberland Ranger District, Gladie Cultural-Environmental Learning Center: 606-663-8100, tinyurl.com/gladie

Sheltowee Trace

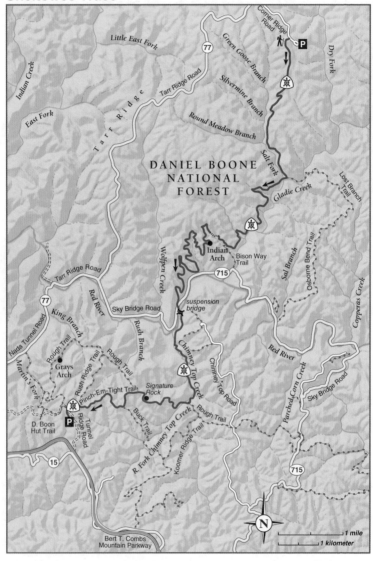

Overview

The Sheltowee Trace, Kentucky's most famous trail, runs on a north–south route for about 270 miles through the length of Kentucky before continuing south into Tennessee. About 17 of those miles cross the length of the Red River Gorge Geological Area and the Clifty Wilderness—with an additional stretch running through Natural Bridge State Resort Park. Parts of this hike, with its famous white turtle blazes, are also among the most popular with hikers and especially backpackers. On the other hand, some stretches will feel positively remote.

The southernmost stretch of the trail follows Whittleton Branch Trail (see Hike 15, page 98). This hike covers 14 miles of the Sheltowee from the Corner Ridge Trailhead in the north to the Pinch-Em-Tight Trailhead in the south. This stretch of the Sheltowee Trace contains not only some of the most rigorous hiking in the Gorge but also some of the best scenery. The route passes a number of large creeks, including Gladie and Chimney Top, and also three of the most famous rock formations: Indian Arch, the Indian Staircase, and Signature Rock, all open to exploration with care. The trail crosses the Red River over a long suspension bridge. The forest, too, is dense along the way.

Because of its length, this trail is best done by shuttle, beginning at the Corner Ridge Trailhead and descending to the Red River,

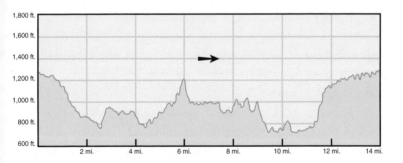

and from there climbing Pinch-Em-Tight Ridge back to Tunnel Ridge Road. Its length also makes this an excellent opportunity for back-packing, and the sheer amount of water along the trail—there is an abundance of creeks—makes it a consistent one.

Route Details

The northernmost stretch of the Sheltowee Trace begins at the Corner Ridge Trailhead, at the dead end of Corner Ridge Road—also part of the trace. The initial trail is actually an old logging road; watch for the old wooden posts along the way, not to mention the occasional sign and culvert. Expect this part of the trail to be wide and easy but also trampled by horses. The old road heads south and descends gradually for 2.8 miles to a junction with Lost Branch Trail and a confluence of Gladie Creek and Salt Fork. At the junction sign for Lost Branch, go to the right, downhill and toward the creek. At Gladie Creek, the trail fords the small Salt Fork; pay attention here, as the path is easy to lose. Watch for a white arrow blazed on a tree, pointing to the right; here the Sheltowee ascends the hill, paralleling Gladie Creek.

The Sheltowee continues 2.3 miles beyond this ford, crossing several other side creeks—Garrett, Hale, and Klaber Branches—as it passes through a seldom-traveled section of the Clifty Wilderness before leaving the wilderness area and reaching the Bison Way junction. At this Y-junction, go right and uphill. This next stretch of trail is, without a doubt, one of the most popular day hikes in the entire region, as it passes several notable destinations. On a busy weekend, expect to meet many hikers, if not large groups. At this point, you have traveled 5.1 miles.

From here, it's a short hike to one of the most popular destinations in the Red River Gorge: the Indian Staircase, a water-carved staircase that ascends a sandstone cliff overlooking a forested box canyon. From the junction with Bison Way Trail, follow the Sheltowee 0.3 mile, crossing two small creeks. Watch for two side trails to the right: one will be clearly marked as CLOSED by the U.S. Forest Service, but the second is the actual spur trail. Follow this trail up a narrow ridge to a cliff. Head up a notch and emerge at the sandstone base of the Indian Staircase. From here, be extremely careful, and do *not* attempt to climb the steps in wet weather. For an added bonus, you can find KY Arch 80 by going a bit to the right along the base of the sandstone cliff. If you're not in the mood for climbing, the view here from the base of the steps is enough.

Return to the trace and go right, continuing another 0.2 mile to a stairway, atop which lies Indian Arch. From here, the Sheltowee Trace weaves in and out of drainages, rising and falling along scenic cliffs and rock shelters for 3.4 miles, descending to KY 715. Cross the road and descend the hill to the obvious suspension bridge over the Red River. At this point, you have hiked 10 miles.

A trail on the northern shore of the Red River is worth exploring; it goes west 0.4 mile along the bank to a trailhead parking area. On a sunny weekend you will find many campsites here. Cross the Red River on the long bridge, and then follow the river downstream to the right before turning uphill along Chimney Top Creek. The next 1.5 miles follow the creek and ford both it and a side creek before meeting the Rough Trail. Go right on the combination Sheltowee Trace/Rough Trail for 1 mile, fording Chimney Top Creek for the last time, then quickly crossing the Right Fork of Chimney Top before beginning the long climb upward. In a little less than a mile, the trail quickly gains about 400 feet in elevation, crossing the edge of a burn and reaching Signature Rock. This is a great place to rest and take in the scenery.

Continue a short distance past Signature Rock to a junction with Pinch-Em-Tight Trail. Here the Rough Trail goes right; instead, go left to stay on Sheltowee Trace. In another 0.4 mile, stay right at a junction with the Buck Trail. Follow Pinch-Em-Tight Trail for 0.7 mile, all the way to Tunnel Ridge Road (passing the junction for Rush Ridge Trail on the right), crossing this dirt road to continue on Pinch-Em-Tight Trail the remaining 0.3 mile to the trailhead parking.

Directions

For the Corner Ridge Trailhead, take Exit 33 off Bert T. Combs Mountain Parkway and go north on KY 11 to the junction of KY 15. Go left on KY 15 for 1.5 miles to KY 77. Go right on KY 77 and travel 11.8 miles (the road goes through Nada Tunnel, crosses the Red River, and continues past the Frenchburg Job Corps Conservation Center). Turn right on Corner Ridge Road, following it 1 mile to its end at a small parking area.

For the Pinch-Em-Tight Trailhead, take Exit 33 off Bert T. Combs Mountain Parkway and go north on KY 11 to the junction with KY 15. Go right on KY 15 for 1.5 miles. In 3.5 miles turn left onto gravel Tunnel Ridge Road (Forest Service Road 39). After 0.7 mile turn left into the parking lot for the Pinch-Em-Tight Trailhead.

Silvermine Arch and Cliff Trail

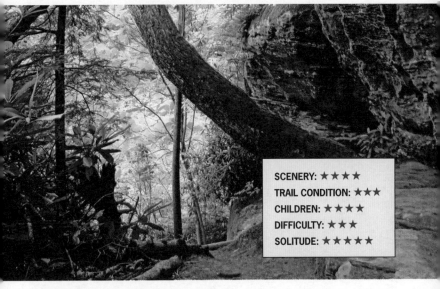

SCENERY: ★ ★ ★ ★
TRAIL CONDITION: ★ ★ ★
CHILDREN: ★ ★ ★ ★
DIFFICULTY: ★ ★ ★
SOLITUDE: ★ ★ ★ ★ ★

CLIFFS LINE THE SILVERMINE ARCH TRAIL.

GPS TRAILHEAD COORDINATES: *Silvermine Arch Trailhead* N37° 46.888' W83° 38.164'

DISTANCE & CONFIGURATION: 1.5-mile out-and-back to Silvermine Arch, plus 1.6-mile out-and-back on the Cliff Trail

HIKING TIME: 2 hours

HIGHLIGHTS: Cliffs, rock formations, viewpoints, and Silvermine Arch

ELEVATION: 1,245' at the trailhead, descending to 1,063'

ACCESS: Open 24/7; vehicle pass required for overnight parking

MAPS: USGS *Slade* and *Pomeroyton;* USFS *Red River Gorge Geological Area*

FACILITIES: Restrooms and water available at campground

WHEELCHAIR ACCESS: None

COMMENTS: Early parts of this trail are nearly obscured by poison ivy; take care in the beginning section through the campground, or, if it suits you, follow the roads through the campground to an alternate trailhead at campsite 35. Cliffs are especially precarious atop and around Silvermine Arch, so use extreme caution.

CONTACTS: Daniel Boone National Forest, Cumberland Ranger District, Gladie Cultural-Environmental Learning Center: 606-663-8100, tinyurl.com/gladie

Silvermine Arch and Cliff Trail

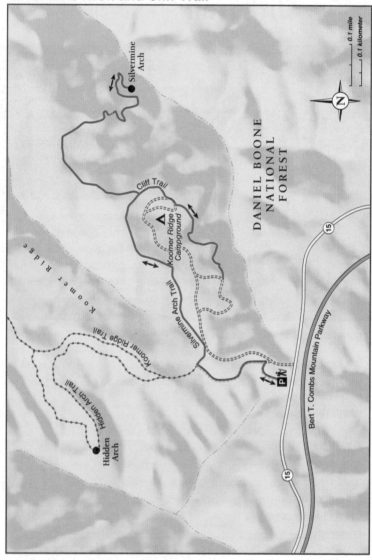

Overview

If you happen to be camping at Koomer Ridge Campground, there's really no reason not to hike the trails that begin in the campground itself. They make a great early-morning or late-afternoon hike for families, especially given their relatively short lengths. The longer of the two descends the cliffs to Silvermine Arch. This underappreciated trail offers not only solitude and quiet but also an opportunity to explore a wondrous grotto surrounding the arch, topped with thickets of rhododendrons and views into a nearby ravine and the imposing cliffs above it. Setting out from Koomer Ridge Campground, this short and fairly easy trail goes down a long staircase and continues to fall through a forest of poplars and hemlocks to an extraordinary and virtually unpopulated arch, punctuated by the sounds of trickling water. Connected to the Silvermine Arch Trail, the Cliff Trail is a designated National Recreation Trail despite its length. Only 0.8 mile long, it follows a sheer cliff along the edge of the campground and provides great photo opportunities.

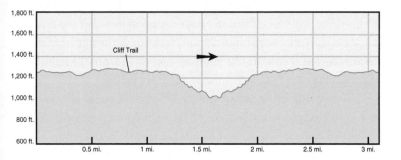

Route Details

Silvermine Arch is an eroded cliffline, a grotto wet with dripping water that can make the ground muddy but the area under the arch pleasantly cool. You're afforded opportunities to explore, but you should do so with the utmost care. A number of deadly cliffs sit near the arch, especially from the top of it. It's probably best to stay below the arch and play.

The trailhead for Silvermine Arch is an easy 500 feet from the parking lot, adjacent to the campground host's site. Follow this combination trail for Koomer Ridge, Hidden Arch, and Silvermine Arch for 0.2 mile through the campground to a junction, then go right, following signs for the Silvermine Arch Trail.

The next 0.2 mile weaves through the campground, passing an amphitheater and crossing a dirt U.S. Forest Service road. Ignore the abundant side trails leading to campsites and stay on the most obvious trail. Eventually, Silvermine Arch Trail intersects the end of the Cliff Trail at 0.6 mile. The Cliff Trail provides an option to lengthen the hike by 1.6 miles; though it is a National Recreation Trail, it nonetheless skips along some domineering cliffs and even provides a small amphitheater where you could spend an hour sitting and contemplating the distant ridges. Consider adding this very easy trail after your hike to Silvermine Arch.

If you're continuing on to Silvermine Arch, go 90 degrees to the left here. The trail soon passes an overgrown meadow before heading into the deeper hardwood forest. At the 1-mile mark, the trail reaches a sweeping overlook at the top of a steep stairway. Take in the sights, but be careful near the edge, as this is a precipitous drop.

A seemingly never-ending staircase descends 79 steps and about 50 feet in elevation into the forested ravine, following closely along jutting rock outcrops. At the end of the trail, about 0.75 mile and 250 feet down from the ridge, you'll reach the dark and dripping grotto of Silvermine Arch, where ferns, rhododendrons, and holly bushes grow profusely. Explore the arch, but beware of the cliffs that surround it. Be prepared to ascend the steep trail to return as you came.

If you do decide to head out on the Cliff Trail, go left at its junction with the Silvermine Arch Trail. The Cliff Trail first meanders through the woods just behind some campsites, emerging onto the road between sites 39 and 41. Follow the road to the left, and the trail will pick up again between sites 36 and 35. Now the trail gets more interesting, following the edge of a steep cliff and passing a number of overlooks, including a small amphitheater—a good place to sit. Stay away from the edge! The trail emerges on one of the campground's loops by site 13.

From here, you have the option of following the trail back to the Silvermine Arch Trail, and then returning as you came by continuing straight on the Silvermine Arch Trail at that junction and heading back to your car, or you can follow the road back. If you opt for the easy way along the road, come off the Cliff Trail by site 13 and follow the road to the right. This will bring you to an intersection by the campground's bathhouse. Go left and follow this road to an intersection by the campground host's quarters. Take a right, then a quick left, and you'll be back at the trailhead parking area.

Directions

From Exit 33 off Bert T. Combs Mountain Parkway, go 0.1 mile north on KY 11 and turn right on KY 15. In 5.1 miles turn left at the sign for Koomer Ridge Campground and immediately turn left onto a short spur road to the trailhead parking area.

13   Sky Bridge

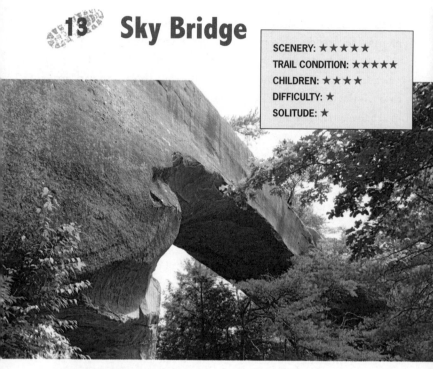

SCENERY: ★ ★ ★ ★ ★
TRAIL CONDITION: ★ ★ ★ ★ ★
CHILDREN: ★ ★ ★
DIFFICULTY: ★
SOLITUDE: ★

CHILDREN IN STROLLERS AND PEOPLE IN WHEELCHAIRS CAN GO AS FAR AS THE SKY BRIDGE ARCH ALONG THIS TRAIL.

GPS TRAILHEAD COORDINATES: *Sky Bridge Recreation Area*
N37° 49.064' W83° 34.937'

DISTANCE & CONFIGURATION: 0.8-mile loop

HIGHLIGHTS: An impressive arch, panoramic views, and an easy paved trail

HIKING TIME: 1 hour

ELEVATION: 1,135' at the trailhead, descending to 982'

ACCESS: Open 24/7, except during winter storms; vehicle pass required for overnight parking

MAPS: USGS *Pomeroyton;* USFS *Red River Gorge Geological Area*

FACILITIES: Restrooms and picnic area

WHEELCHAIR ACCESS: Yes; strollers can be taken as far as Sky Bridge, but past that is not recommended.

COMMENTS: Dangerous cliffs are present and should be avoided, especially by children.

CONTACTS: Daniel Boone National Forest, Cumberland Ranger District, Gladie Cultural-Environmental Learning Center: 606-663-8100, tinyurl.com/gladie

Overview

Of all the trails in the Red River Gorge, this short path is likely the most heavily used of them all. Granted, the drive alone is stunning: the access road, as well as the trail, stretches along a ridge dividing the deep ravine of Swift Camp Creek from Devil's Canyon. And the arch is one of the most picturesque and heavily photographed in the region. Because of this, and the fact that this is one of the few paved trails to such a landmark, you can expect, especially on weekends, a heavy influx of visitors, children, and even buses. Nevertheless, you shouldn't let this stop you.

Sky Bridge is exactly as it sounds: the trail crosses the arch, offering truly stunning views of the surrounding gorges, forests, and rock formations. Surprisingly, most people walk to the arch, take a few pictures, and turn right around. But the trail goes on, forming a loop that will take you below the arch for the most amazing sight: Sky Bridge is also technically a double arch, with one smoothed and rounded pillar making two windows over Devil's Canyon. This is a great place to bring kids, as the trail is easy and the scenery impressive, but be very aware of the dangers. Sky Bridge has seen its share of tragedies over the years—*stay on the trail, and don't go near the edge.*

Route Details

From the parking lot, follow either the road or the paved path to the north end of the picnic area, toward the loop end of the road. At the sign, follow the paved Sky Bridge Trail a mere 0.2 mile to the top of the arch. The trail descends very gradually and easily, part of the reason this trail is so popular and noticeably overused. There is an overlook at the start of the span, but the trail continues over it. Be especially aware of the height of the arch and stay away from the edge. From the top of the arch you will have unimpeded views. To the west is Devil's Canyon, with a number of cliffs and rock formations prominently displayed among the trees. To the east, Swift Camp Creek's gorge dominates the landscape.

Sky Bridge

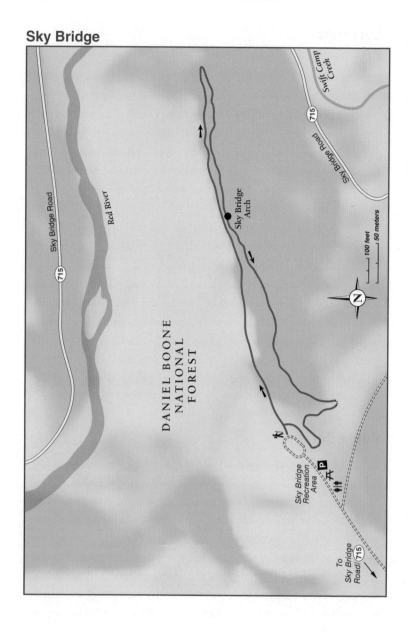

To continue on the loop, cross the arch and continue on the trail. The path here is lined with stone walls and iron railings. Descend a set of stairs about 60 feet. The trail doubles back to the right and heads south, as it returns to the parking lot. At 0.4 mile the trail ascends a series of steps and returns to the arch, this time from the base. Notice that there are actually two arches here: the large span and a smaller one to the right, both of which offer vistas west to Devil's Canyon. Notice, also, the sheer amount of damage done to the sandstone by the incessant name-carving from years past. Follow the cliffs to a long stairway at 0.6 mile. The trail climbs a bit steeper before it returns to the parking lot.

Directions

From Exit 40 off Bert T. Combs Mountain Parkway, go right on KY 15/KY 715 for 1 mile, and then follow KY 715 to the right for 4.9 miles to the Sky Bridge Recreation Area spur road. Go left for 0.8 mile to the parking area, at the road's end.

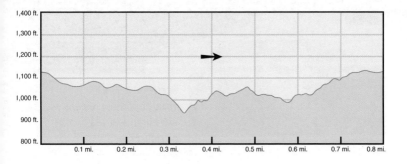

14 Whistling Arch

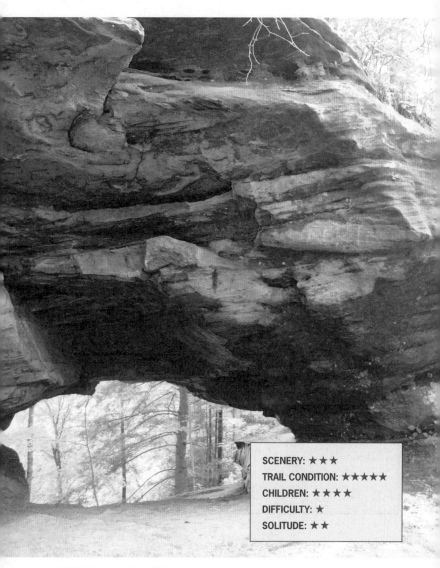

SCENERY: ★ ★ ★
TRAIL CONDITION: ★ ★ ★ ★ ★
CHILDREN: ★ ★ ★ ★
DIFFICULTY: ★
SOLITUDE: ★ ★

WHISTLING ARCH FRAMES A GORGEOUS VISTA.

GPS TRAILHEAD COORDINATES: Whistling Arch Trailhead N37° 48.474' W83° 35.412'

DISTANCE & CONFIGURATION: 0.4-mile out-and-back

HIGHLIGHTS: Cliffs, rock formations, and a small arch with good views

HIKING TIME: 0.5 hour

ELEVATION: 1,140' at the trailhead, with no significant elevation gain or loss

ACCESS: Open 24/7; vehicle pass required for overnight parking

MAPS: USGS Pomeroyton; USFS Red River Gorge Geological Area

FACILITIES: None

WHEELCHAIR ACCESS: None

COMMENTS: Dangerous cliffs are present and should be avoided, especially by children.

CONTACTS: Daniel Boone National Forest, Cumberland Ranger District, Gladie Cultural-Environmental Learning Center: 606-663-8100, tinyurl.com/gladie

Overview

A very easy stroll through the forest for everyone, including families, this trail leads to an impressive cliff where Whistling Arch is set. Why it is named that is anyone's guess, though it may be on account of the wail of wind that may come up from the ravines. Visit in spring, when the flowers are blooming, or fall, when autumn colors flare along the trail. Though it is possible to scramble to the top of the rock formation, do so with extreme caution.

Route Details

From the parking lot, Whistling Arch Trail heads into the piney woods. About 700 feet down the trail, you'll arrive at an unmarked junction with a trail leading right. Stay to the left, following the more obvious path.

After only 0.2 mile the trail arrives at the cliff and a substantial rock shelter on the right. Note also the extreme drop-off at this point. At first glance, the arch will not be visible. The arch is visible in one of two ways: either by going off the trail to the right toward the cliff a short distance (the rock-shelter floor is mostly sand and has sturdy flat sections) or by continuing on the trail past the formation and turning around to look. The second way will make the arch more

Whistling Arch

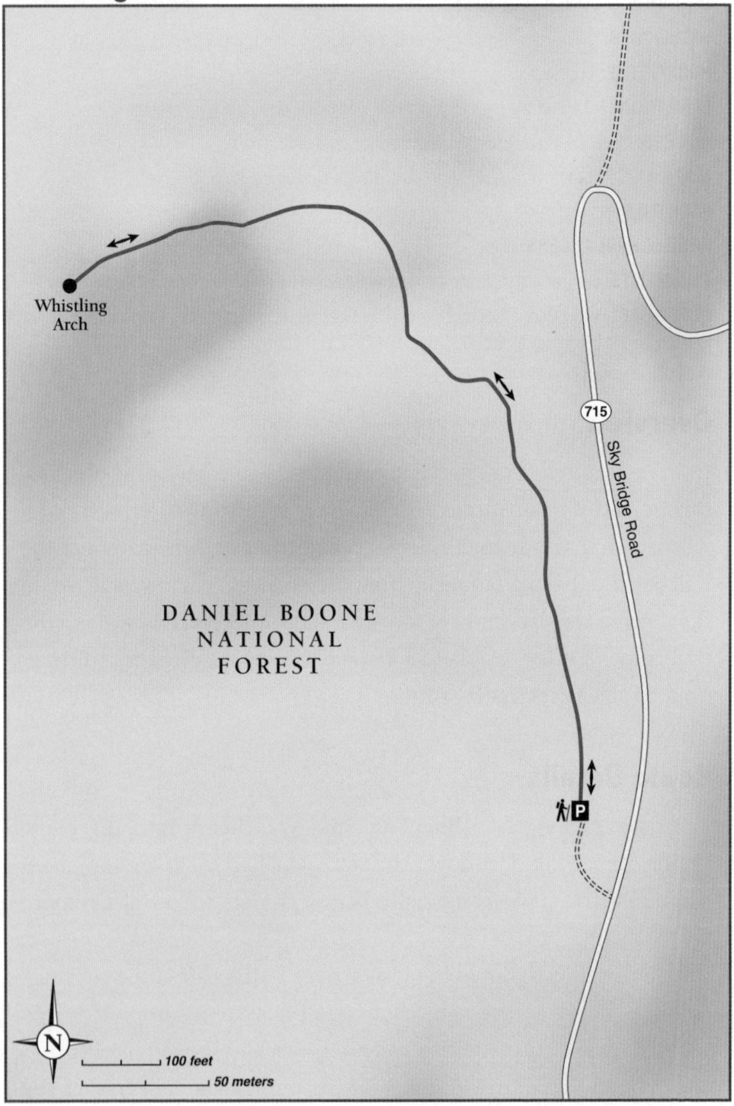

Whistling
Arch

715

Sky Bridge Road

DANIEL BOONE
NATIONAL
FOREST

N

100 feet

50 meters

prominent, framing the view of the gorges beyond. The U.S. Forest Service calls this kind of arch a buttress-type formation.

A bit past the arch, the trail ends, looking out over Parched Corn Creek drainage. A number of side trails scurry up the cliffs, but disregard them, as they are dangerous. You are likely to find this trail unpopulated, so enjoy the quiet. Return as you came.

Directions

From Exit 40 off Bert T. Combs Mountain Parkway, go right on KY 15/KY 715 for 1 mile, and then follow KY 715 right for 4.7 miles to the Whistling Arch Trailhead parking area, on the left. The trail begins just across the road.

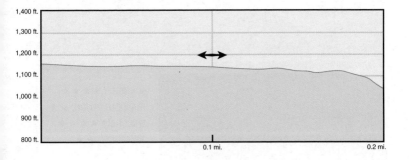

15 Whittleton Arch

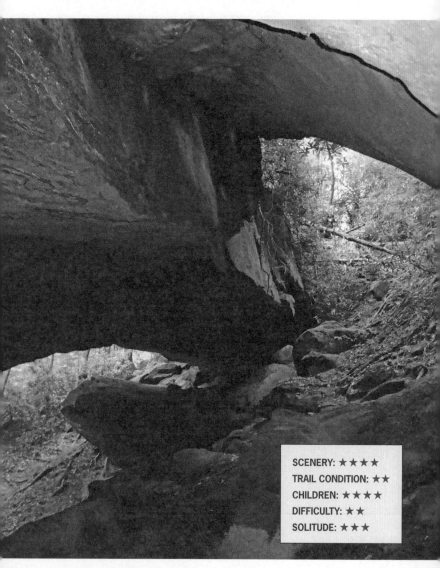

SCENERY: ★★★★
TRAIL CONDITION: ★★
CHILDREN: ★★★★
DIFFICULTY: ★★
SOLITUDE: ★★★

VIEW BENEATH WHITTLETON ARCH

GPS TRAILHEAD COORDINATES: *Whittleton Campground* N37° 46.811' W83° 40.492'

DISTANCE & CONFIGURATION: 4.4-mile out-and-back

HIGHLIGHTS: Creekside walk along a historic railway grade, spring wildflowers, and Whittleton Arch

HIKING TIME: 3 hours

ELEVATION: 764' at the trailhead, ascending to 1,333'

ACCESS: No dogs are allowed on trails in Natural Bridge State Resort Park.

MAPS: USGS *Slade;* Natural Bridge State Resort Park Trail Guide; USFS *Red River Gorge Geological Area*

FACILITIES: Restrooms and water in campground

WHEELCHAIR ACCESS: None

COMMENTS: Dangerous cliffs are present and should be avoided, especially by children.

CONTACTS: Natural Bridge State Resort Park: 606-663-2214 or 800-325-1710, parks. ky.gov/parks/resortparks/natural-bridge; Daniel Boone National Forest, Cumberland Ranger District, Gladie Cultural-Environmental Learning Center: 606-663-8100, tinyurl.com/gladie

Overview

Whittleton Branch is one of the best creeks to hike beside in the Gorge region. Depending on the time of year, it may be overflowing or languid, loud or quiet, but either way, this creek—with its streamside stroll and wooden footbridges—is one of the most picturesque of all the creekside hikes. The added bonus is that a short side trail leads to one of the most well-known formations in the Gorge, Whittleton Arch, which is the largest arch by mass in the Gorge area. Not quite as dramatic as, say, nearby Natural Bridge, it nonetheless has its own charm. It is actually more like a massive rock shelter with part of its roof worn away. After a good rain, a waterfall plunges over the shelf, falling into a creek that slips off into a ravine. There's also abundant history here: the upper stretch of Whittleton Branch Trail clearly shows its former use as a railroad grade, even making use of some of the original railroad ties to cross wet areas. This hike follows the Sheltowee Trace, which crosses the state of Kentucky north to south. This 2-mile path is part of an impressive stretch marching through the Red River Gorge Geological Area and Natural Bridge State Resort Park. A very short section of this hike follows the road

Whittleton Arch

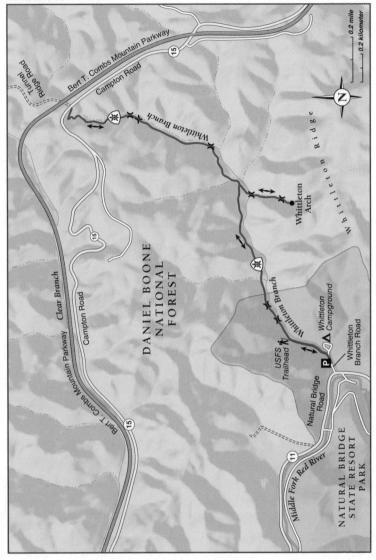

through Whittleton Campground, clearly labeled by the white diamond blazes and the turtle-shell blaze of the Sheltowee Trace.

Route Details

From the parking area, follow the Sheltowee Trace north through the campground. As it does in many places, the trail actually follows the road here. At the end of the pavement, the trailhead sign for Whittleton Branch Trail is clearly visible. From here, you leave the state park and enter the Daniel Boone National Forest.

The lower half of this trail is level and easy, crossing the creek on wooden footbridges—a rarity in the Red River Gorge. House-size boulders litter the creekbed, and the forest is dense and rich with low-elevation hardwood trees. The trail crosses and recrosses Whittleton Branch several times.

At 0.7 mile the stream actually disappears. This is due to the region's karst geology, part of which involves the weathering of limestone, producing caves and sinkholes. The creek here, in other words, actually runs underground. For the rest of the trail, the creek will periodically reappear and disappear again. The trail leaves the creek and climbs the hillside—repair from a washout of a few years earlier.

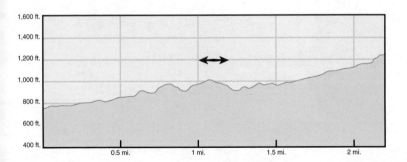

At 0.8 mile you'll reach the junction with Whittleton Arch Trail on the right. To visit the arch, turn here and cross the footbridge.

The trail to the arch climbs steadily, gaining 100 feet over sometimes muddy and rocky ground, for 0.2 mile, following a creek on the left. At the top of the ravine, depending on the time of year, you may hear a waterfall. The trail emerges in a massive amphitheater-like grotto. The arch is not evident until you climb into the massive rock shelter. The formation of this "arch" occurred when the back of the shelter was worn away by water; this phenomenon is called a waterfall step arch. The dusty floor, covered in large boulders, makes a cool and pleasant spot to rest.

To continue on the Whittleton Branch Trail to KY 15, head back down Whittleton Arch Trail for 0.2 mile to the junction. Now go right on the Whittleton Branch Trail. From here, the forest canopy thins a bit, and the trail may become noticeably hotter. You may also notice that this section is not as frequently traveled as the lower section.

FOOTBRIDGE OVER WHITTLETON BRANCH

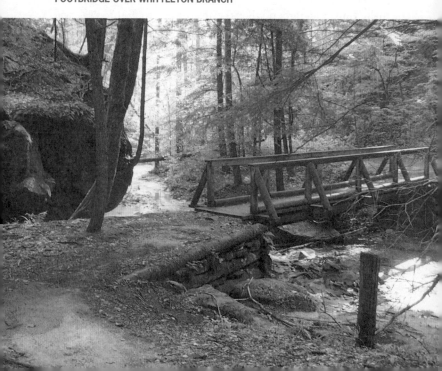

Over the next 1.2 miles, the trail climbs gradually toward KY 15. The path crosses the creek, and for a long distance it stays mostly on the east side of the creek. Along this route are several waterfalls, a number of hidden rock shelters, and, at 1.25 miles, a very muddy spot that is lined with the old, original railroad ties. Nearing the end of the trail, you will begin to hear traffic. The final stretch of trail leaves the creek behind and switchbacks up to the road.

The top of the trail is well marked, lying directly across from gravel Tunnel Ridge Road. The route of the Sheltowee Trace follows this road over the bridge (which crosses Bert T. Combs Mountain Parkway) before heading again into the woods. This is a convenient spot to leave a vehicle for a shuttle, as the distance is not terribly far from Whittleton Campground. But this trail still makes a fine out-and-back hike, and the return, only 2 miles to the lower trailhead, is easy and downhill.

Directions

From Exit 33 off Bert T. Combs Mountain Parkway, drive south on KY 11 for 2.2 miles to the entrance of Whittleton Campground. Turn left into the campground and park on the right in a small lot just beyond the woodshed. Follow the road into the campground to its end, where the trailhead is clearly marked. A shuttle is possible by leaving a vehicle on KY 15 at the junction with Tunnel Ridge Road. Park along the side of KY 15 near the trail sign directly across from Tunnel Ridge Road.

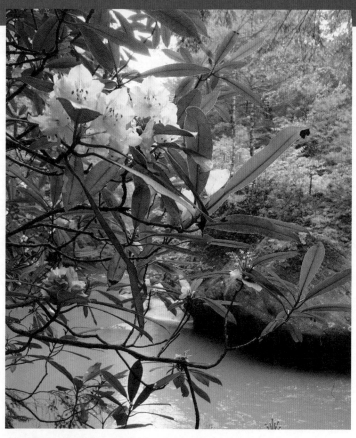

RHODODENDRONS LINE SWIFT CAMP CREEK. *(Hike 19, page 121)*

16 SHELTOWEE TRACE–BISON WAY LOOP 105

17 SHELTOWEE TRACE–OSBORNE BEND LOOP 110

18 SWIFT CAMP CREEK TRAIL 115

19 SWIFT CAMP CREEK–WILDCAT LOOP 121

20 TOWER ROCK 127

21 TURTLE BACK ARCH 131

Sheltowee Trace–Bison Way Loop

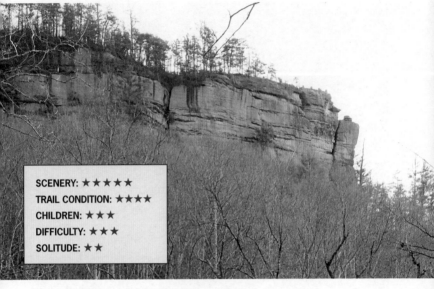

SCENERY: ★ ★ ★ ★ ★
TRAIL CONDITION: ★ ★ ★ ★
CHILDREN: ★ ★ ★
DIFFICULTY: ★ ★ ★
SOLITUDE: ★ ★

SANDSTONE RIDGE ABOVE THE INDIAN STAIRCASE

GPS TRAILHEAD COORDINATES: *Bison Way Trailhead* N37° 50.210' W83° 36.565'
Sheltowee Trace Suspension Bridge Trailhead N37° 49.380' W83° 37.682'

DISTANCE & CONFIGURATION: 5.3-mile point-to-point

HIGHLIGHTS: Numerous arches and cliff formations, rugged forest trails, and a swinging bridge over the Red River

HIKING TIME: 5 hours

ELEVATION: 750' at the trailhead, with a gain of 463'

ACCESS: Open 24/7; vehicle pass required for overnight parking

MAPS: USGS *Pomeroyton;* USFS *Red River Gorge Geological Area*

FACILITIES: Restrooms

WHEELCHAIR ACCESS: None

COMMENTS: This hike is best done as a shuttle, beginning at the Bison Way Trailhead and ending at the Suspension Bridge Trailhead, both on KY 715. Dangerous cliffs are present and should be avoided, especially by children.

CONTACTS: Daniel Boone National Forest, Cumberland Ranger District, Gladie Cultural-Environmental Learning Center: 606-663-8100, tinyurl.com/gladie

Sheltowee Trace–Bison Way Loop

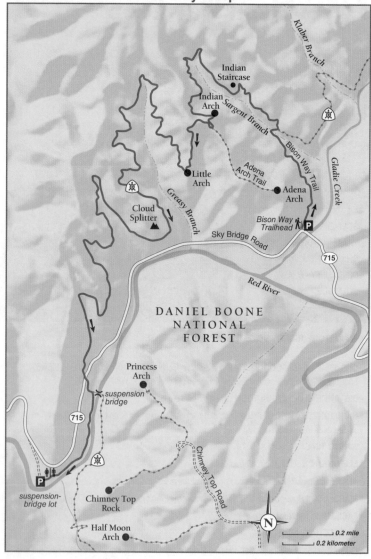

Overview

It is entirely possible that of all the trails the Red River Gorge has to offer, this one is the most popular. Two reasons quickly come to mind: the Indian Staircase, a water-scoured formation up a steep sandstone cliff that rewards with a commanding view, and Indian Arch, to which the trail climbs. Other notable formations, such as the Adena Arch and Cloud Splitter, lie hidden back in the forest. The forest, too, is dense and seems nearly impenetrable at times. If hiking the entire stretch of the Sheltowee Trace through the Red River Gorge seems daunting, this shorter hike would be the best introduction to what the Sheltowee has to offer. You could start at either end and make a return trip to the vehicle, but it's far more worthwhile to shuttle between two trailheads, starting at the easier entrance at the Bison Way Trailhead, and make this a full exploration of one of the best parts of the Sheltowee Trace.

Route Details

The hike begins at Bison Way Trailhead, which lies just above wide and languid Gladie Creek, near the Gladie Cultural-Environmental Learning Center. From the parking lot, head into the forest on the mostly level Bison Way Trail 210. This is the easiest part of the hike;

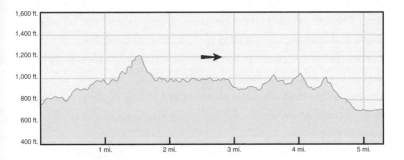

the Bison Way Trail is really no more than an access trail to the Shel-towee Trace. Follow it for 0.8 mile, climbing steadily but easily up a small gully before finally descending a set of wooden stairs to a crossing of Sargent Branch. Just beyond the creek you will arrive at the junction with the Sheltowee Trace. Go left and uphill on the Shel-towee, prominently marked with both white diamonds and white turtle blazes. (*Sheltowee,* meaning "turtle," was the name given to Daniel Boone upon his capture by the Shawnee.)

From here, it's a fairly short hike to one of the most popular destinations in the Red River Gorge: the Indian Staircase, a water-carved staircase that ascends a sandstone cliff overlooking a forested box canyon. From the junction with the Bison Way Trail, follow the Sheltowee 0.3 mile, crossing two small creeks. Watch for two side trails to the right: one will be clearly marked as CLOSED by the U.S. Forest Service, but the second is the actual spur trail. Follow this spur trail up a narrow ridge to a cliff. Head up a notch in the cliff and emerge at the sandstone base of the Indian Staircase. From here, be careful, and do *not* attempt to climb the steps in wet weather. For an added bonus, you can find the KY Arch 80 by going a bit to the right along the base of the sandstone cliff. If you're not in the mood for climbing, the view here from the base of the steps is enough.

Return to the trace, turn right, and continue another 0.2 mile, climbing out of the box canyon to a stairway, atop which lies Indian Arch. The arch, at the highest elevation of the hike and the 1.5-mile mark, makes an excellent resting spot, as most of the difficult climb-ing is over by this point. If you continue on, the trail soon sharply descends a series of sandstone switchbacks. Watch for a side trail on the left where the path turns sharply right at one of these switch-backs—peek around the corner and you will see one of the smallest arches in the Gorge.

From here, the Sheltowee Trace rises and falls along scenic cliffs and rock shelters for 3.4 miles, descending to KY 715. Along the way, the trail also coils like a snake as it weaves in and out of drainages, including a large one named Greasy Branch, and circles the massive

Cloud Splitter Rock before dropping into the river valley. At the highway, cross the road and descend the hill to the obvious suspension bridge over the Red River. On a sunny day, you're sure to find a number of people playing on the bridge, swinging it as far as they can.

Just before the bridge, a side trail leads to the right. Follow this trail 0.4 mile to the Suspension Bridge Trailhead to complete the shuttle. To make this hike into a loop, walk 1.8 miles along paved KY 715.

Directions

To reach the Sheltowee Trace Suspension Bridge Trailhead, start from Bert T. Combs Mountain Parkway, take Exit 33, and go north on KY 11 to the junction with KY 15. Go west on KY 15 for 1.5 miles, and then turn right on KY 77. Follow KY 77 for 5.3 miles to an intersection with KY 715. Go straight on KY 715 for 1.6 miles to the trailhead, on the right.

To reach the Bison Way Trailhead, follow the directions above, going an additional 1.8 miles to a parking area on the left, just before the Gladie Creek Bridge.

Sheltowee Trace— Osborne Bend Loop

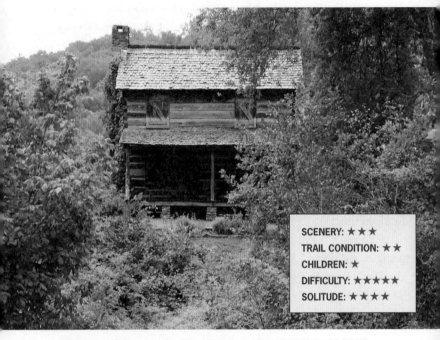

SCENERY: ★ ★ ★
TRAIL CONDITION: ★ ★
CHILDREN: ★
DIFFICULTY: ★ ★ ★ ★ ★
SOLITUDE: ★ ★ ★ ★

THE GLADIE CABIN, A LATE 19TH-CENTURY RECONSTRUCTED LOG HOME

GPS TRAILHEAD COORDINATES: *Bison Way Trailhead* N37° 50.210' W83° 36.565'

DISTANCE & CONFIGURATION: 8.7-mile loop

HIKING TIME: 5.5 hours

ELEVATION: 750' at the trailhead, with total elevation change of 542'

ACCESS: Open 24/7; vehicle pass required for overnight parking

MAPS: USGS *Pomeroyton;* USFS *Red River Gorge Geological Area*

FACILITIES: Restroom

WHEELCHAIR ACCESS: None

COMMENTS: Salt Fork Creek requires fording, which can be difficult after heavy rains or in springtime. Lost Branch Trail 239 is an extremely damaged horse trail and can be very muddy.

CONTACTS: Daniel Boone National Forest, Cumberland Ranger District, Gladie Cultural-Environmental Learning Center: 606-663-8100, tinyurl.com/gladie

Overview

The Clifty Wilderness, along the eastern border of the Red River Gorge Geological Area, is one of only two designated wilderness areas in the state of Kentucky. Remarkably, it is nearly devoid of people. The famous Sheltowee Trace crosses the northern range of the Clifty, descending to the Red River and crossing the Red River Gorge Geological Area. This loop hike, difficult but exhilarating, accesses the Sheltowee from Bison Way Trail 210, then climbs into the wilderness area, roughly following the canyon of Gladie Creek. The loop comes down to the lazy Gladie, crossing it and then setting off on Lost Branch Trail 239, a historical road that is now a rough and damaged horse trail. If you can make it up there, the rest of the loop proves easier, leaving the hoofprints behind and setting off downhill on the Osborne Bend Trail 240. The last leg of the trip follows KY 715 along the Red River, passing several access points and a nice waterfall.

Route Details

From the parking lot, head into the forest on the mostly level Bison Way Trail. Follow this trail 0.8 mile, walking steadily up a small gully and finally descending a set of wooden stairs to a crossing of Sargent Branch. Just beyond the creek you will arrive at the junction with the Sheltowee Trace. Go right on the Sheltowee, prominently marked with both white diamonds and white turtle blazes (*Sheltowee* means "turtle"), following the sign toward Corner Ridge.

The Sheltowee Trace enters a largely conifer forest, following a ridge above Gladie Creek. Though the trail crosses several smaller creeks, Gladie Creek remains far below on the right, but a few vistas will open both to the creek and the surrounding ridges. The route remains fairly steady along the ridge over Gladie Creek and crosses Klaber, Hale, and Garrett Branches before arriving at the confluence of Salt Fork and Gladie Creek, at 3 miles. To continue, you must ford Salt Fork, which, compared with the stream-hopping done along the way, may come as a surprise. This crossing can be

Sheltowee Trace–Osborne Bend Loop

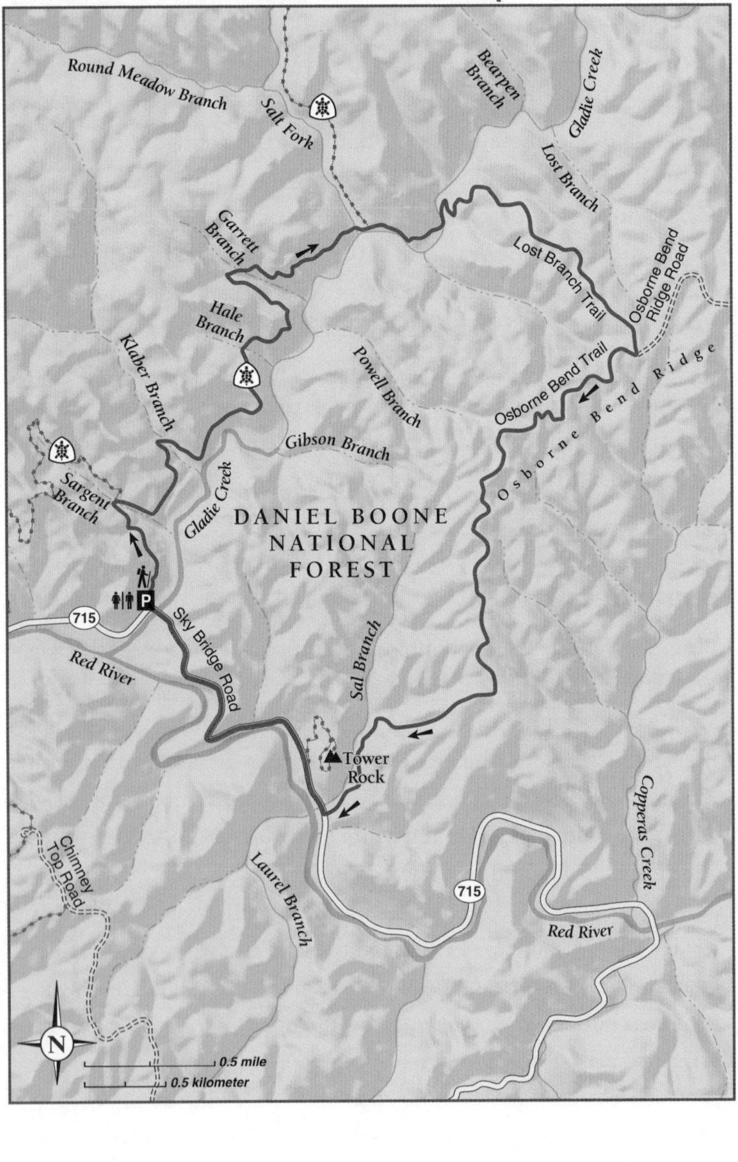

Round Meadow Branch

Bearpen Branch

Gladie Creek

Salt Fork

Lost Branch

Garrett Branch

Lost Branch Trail

Osborne Bend Ridge Road

Hale Branch

Powell Branch

Osborne Bend Trail

Klaber Branch

Gibson Branch

Osborne Bend Ridge

Sargent Branch

DANIEL BOONE
NATIONAL
FOREST

Gladie Creek

715

Sky Bridge Road

Red River

Sal Branch

Tower Rock

Copperas Creek

Chimney Top Road

Laurel Branch

715

Red River

N

0.5 mile

0.5 kilometer

difficult in high water, so be prepared to remove your boots and use hiking poles for balance.

Just beyond the creek lies a jumbled intersection of trails that may be confusing. You are looking for Lost Branch Trail. Beyond Salt Fork, head upward on the trail that goes straight ahead; the connector trails to the left lead to the northbound Sheltowee Trace, which is no longer part of the loop. Over a small hill, you will arrive at a junction and sign for the Lost Branch Trail. Continue straight and to the right, and at 3.3 miles you'll reach the Lost Branch Trail, which parallels Gladie Creek. At a large flat area, watch for a sharp right turn, leading into what looks like a gully, and follow the Lost Branch Trail upward.

From here, the trail gets ugly quickly. Once an old road, this path is now a horse trail—the only horse trail in the whole Red River Gorge area. Unfortunately, it shows. Lost Branch Trail will likely be covered with deep hoofprints and sucking mud, and the whole mess is cobbled with large, loose rocks. To make matters worse, this muddy gully is breathtakingly steep. The trail climbs 450 feet over the course of 1 mile before leveling out on the top of Osborne Bend Ridge.

From here, things get easier, at least for a while. Lost Branch Trail follows this ridge to the east until it meets the Osborne Bend Trail at 4.7 miles. Follow the Osborne Bend Trail to the right. This

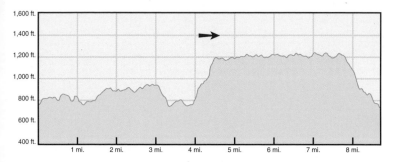

trail, too, will stay high along the ridge for a time. At 6.5 miles the Osborne Bend Trail begins a steep descent back to the highway and the Red River, dropping more than 500 feet in less than a mile. Near the bottom, Sal Branch will be visible to the right. The path at this point is unmaintained, muddy, and rocky. The trail will pass a couple of concrete bunkers of unknown origin and then reach its end on KY 715 at 7.2 miles.

To complete the loop, head to the right and walk west an easy 1.5 miles along the paved highway, which parallels the Red River. The river has several access points, and it's possible to see boaters gliding by. On the north side of the highway, watch for a pretty waterfall, and just before reaching the Bison Way Trailhead, look to the left to see the historical Gladie Cabin set back on a rise beyond a field. Cross the bridge over Gladie Creek and return to your car at the trailhead, on the right.

Directions

From Exit 40 off Bert T. Combs Mountain Parkway, go right on KY 15/KY 715 for 1 mile, and then follow KY 715 right for 10.3 miles to the Bison Way Trailhead on the right, just beyond the bridge over Gladie Creek.

18 Swift Camp Creek Trail

SCENERY: ★ ★ ★ ★
TRAIL CONDITION: ★ ★
CHILDREN: ★ ★ ★
DIFFICULTY: ★ ★ ★
SOLITUDE: ★ ★ ★ ★

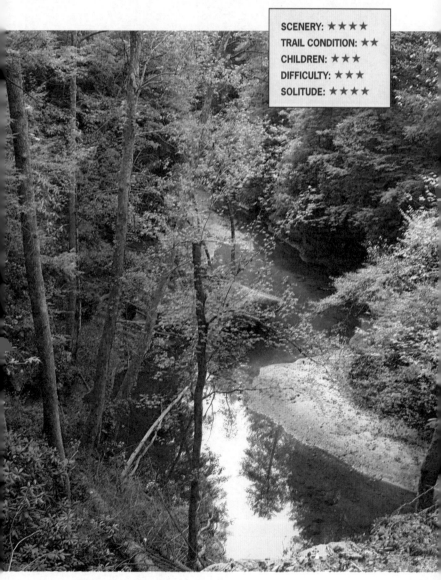

HELL'S KITCHEN IS A NARROW SLOT CANYON IN SWIFT CAMP CREEK.

115

Swift Camp Creek Trail

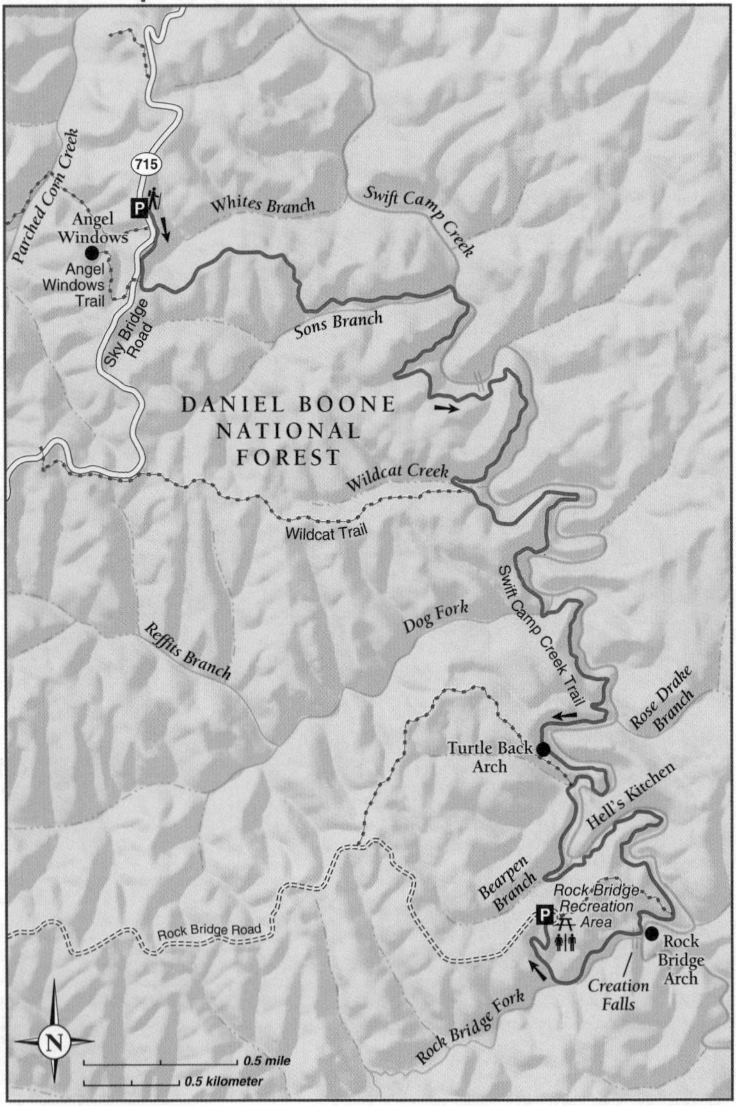

DANIEL BOONE
NATIONAL
FOREST

Parched Corn Creek

715

Angel
Windows

Angel
Windows
Trail

Sky Bridge Road

Whites Branch

Swift Camp Creek

Sons Branch

Wildcat Creek

Wildcat Trail

Reffits Branch

Dog Fork

Swift Camp Creek Trail

Rose Drake
Branch

Turtle Back
Arch

Hell's Kitchen

Bearpen
Branch

Rock Bridge
Recreation
Area

Rock
Bridge
Arch

Rock Bridge Road

Creation
Falls

Rock Bridge Fork

N

0.5 mile

0.5 kilometer

GPS TRAILHEAD COORDINATES: *Rough Trail and Swift Camp Creek Trailhead*
N37° 48.110' W83° 35.451' *Rock Bridge Recreation Area* N37° 46.208' W83° 34.008'

DISTANCE & CONFIGURATION: 7.6-mile point-to-point

HIGHLIGHTS: Backpacking opportunities, exploration points of Swift Camp Creek and
Hell's Kitchen, and Rock Bridge Arch

HIKING TIME: 5 hours

ELEVATION: 1,169' at the trailhead, descending to 752'

ACCESS: Open 24/7; vehicle pass required for overnight parking

MAPS: USGS *Pomeroyton;* USFS *Red River Gorge Geological Area*

FACILITIES: Restrooms at Rock Bridge Recreation Area

WHEELCHAIR ACCESS: None

COMMENTS: This hike is best done as a shuttle, beginning on KY 715 and ending at the
Rock Bridge *Recreation* Area, or else as an extended backpacking trip. Dangerous cliffs are
present and should be avoided, especially by children.

CONTACTS: Daniel Boone National Forest, Cumberland Ranger District, Gladie Cultural-
Environmental Learning Center: 606-663-8100, tinyurl.com/gladie

Overview

One of the best ways to experience the Clifty Wilderness, the Swift
Camp Creek Trail 219 winds along overhanging cliffs and under dense
forests of towering trees. For a stretch, Swift Camp Creek descends
into a nearly inaccessible area called Hell's Kitchen, flowing into deep
grottoes and underneath rock shelters, as well as over waves of sand
and around massive boulders. Be aware that this trail twists and

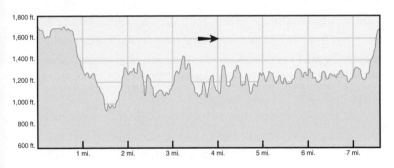

turns with every curve of the creek, which can make this hike seem arduous at times. The trail condition, too, is something to consider: much of it is rugged and narrow and skirts overhanging cliffs.

Route Details

From the combination Rough Trail/Swift Camp Creek Trailhead, follow Swift Camp Creek Trail from the southeast corner of the lot, crossing KY 715 and dropping immediately into the forest. For a short distance the trail parallels the highway, but the path soon leaves the road behind, passing exposed rock formations as it descends. When a side trail intersects from the right near a long rock, continue left at this unmarked junction. When the trail levels, it follows a ridgeline under big oaks and pines for nearly a mile, and then at the 0.8-mile mark it begins a steady descent, dropping nearly 400 feet along Sons Branch, a creek you will likely only hear, as it is densely overgrown with rhododendrons and shrouded in fallen trees.

At the 1.5-mile mark, the trail reaches the confluence of Sons Branch and Swift Camp Creek. Here, the smaller Sons Branch squeezes through and under boulders—watch for the blazes after descending some rock steps that mark this easy ford. Swift Camp Creek is the obvious large stream; note that across the creek a wide landing offers several opportunities for camping. Enjoy the view of the water while you can; from here, the trail begins to climb above the creek, and from this point forward, the creek is mostly inaccessible. Instead, the trail rewards hikers with several rock overhangs, some with seasonal waterfalls, along this stretch. The views over the Swift Camp Creek valley, too, are stunning.

At the 2-mile mark, the trail begins to level out. Just 0.25 mile later, you'll pass a stream beneath a rock shelter. For the next mile, the trail weaves alongside Swift Camp Creek before descending to Wildcat Creek at the 3.3-mile mark. Here the path turns to the right and follows the creek upstream, past a boulder garden, to a crossing where trilliums bloom in the spring. After crossing, the trail curves back downstream to a junction with the Wildcat Trail, which heads uphill to the right.

From here, Swift Camp Creek Trail increases in difficulty. Muddy stretches, narrow paths, steep cliffs, and a nearly constant rise and fall in elevation make this a fairly strenuous hike, which can be tiring for children, not to mention dangerous. At 4.4 miles the trail crosses Dog Fork in one of the loveliest areas of the whole hike; a graceful stream flows lazily past enormous boulders, flowering rhododendrons, and exposed black shale. Campsites are also available in this area, especially on a bench above the creek.

At 5.5 miles a side trail, nearly obscured by rhododendrons, heads right to a perfect campsite and even farther uphill to Turtle Back Arch (see Hike 21, page 131). To the left, a waterfall drops from the cliff into the area known as Hell's Kitchen, which this trail has been following for some distance. Hell's Kitchen is marked by magnificent, albeit inaccessible scenery; access points to the creek are few and far between, so you must be content with the views from on high. The picture, however, is not always perfect—discarded tires and other detritus litter the streambed and are especially visible as water levels drop by late summer and autumn.

At 6 miles the trail slips through a thin gully that is also a creekbed. From here, the remainder of the route is level and dependable, and the path widens. Watch in the last stretch for access points on the left to Swift Camp Creek. Just beyond the 7-mile point, the trail officially ends at the Rock Bridge Trail, the Wilderness Area now left behind. From here, it's worthwhile to see two of the area's best icons, so instead of heading uphill to the right, which leads to the lot at the Rock Bridge Recreation Area, continue straight along Swift Camp Creek for an impressive view of Rock Bridge Arch, a fine way to end the hike.

Expect the last 0.7-mile stretch of trail to be busy. Parts of it are paved, though sometimes that paving is old and deteriorated. Nevertheless, Rock Bridge Arch quickly appears on the left, the only arch of its kind where a creek flows beneath it—hence, the only arch that is a true bridge. Set beneath a stand of towering hemlocks and pines, it makes an ideal rest spot. To complete the journey, continue past the arch, leaving Swift Camp Creek behind and following Rock Bridge Fork to Creation Falls (an overlook is on the left) before heading uphill through a cathedral-like forest to the Rock Bridge Recreation Area.

Directions

To reach the Rough Trail/Swift Camp Creek Trailhead, take Exit 40 off Bert T. Combs Mountain Parkway, go right on KY 15/KY 715 for 1 mile, and then follow KY 715 right for 4.2 miles to the parking area, on the left.

To reach the Rock Bridge Recreation Area, take Exit 40 off Bert T. Combs Mountain Parkway. At the stop sign, go right on KY 15/ KY 715 for 1 mile. Where the roads split in the small community of Pine Ridge, go right (north) on KY 715 for 1 mile, turning right onto gravel Rock Bridge Road (Forest Service Road 24) and continuing 3 miles to the road's end and the parking area, at the Rock Bridge Recreation Area.

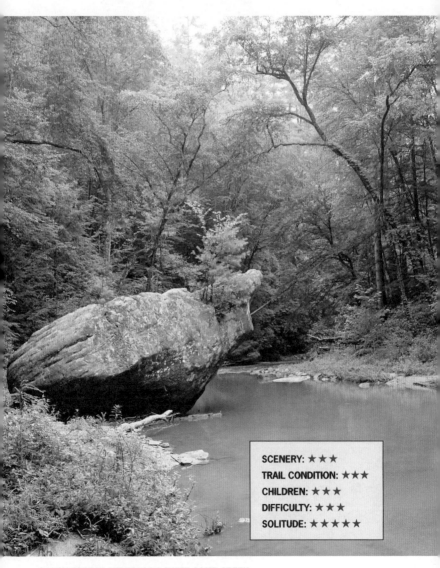

SCENERY: ★ ★ ★
TRAIL CONDITION: ★ ★ ★
CHILDREN: ★ ★ ★
DIFFICULTY: ★ ★ ★
SOLITUDE: ★ ★ ★ ★ ★

A LUSH FOREST SURROUNDS SWIFT CAMP CREEK.

Swift Camp Creek–Wildcat Loop

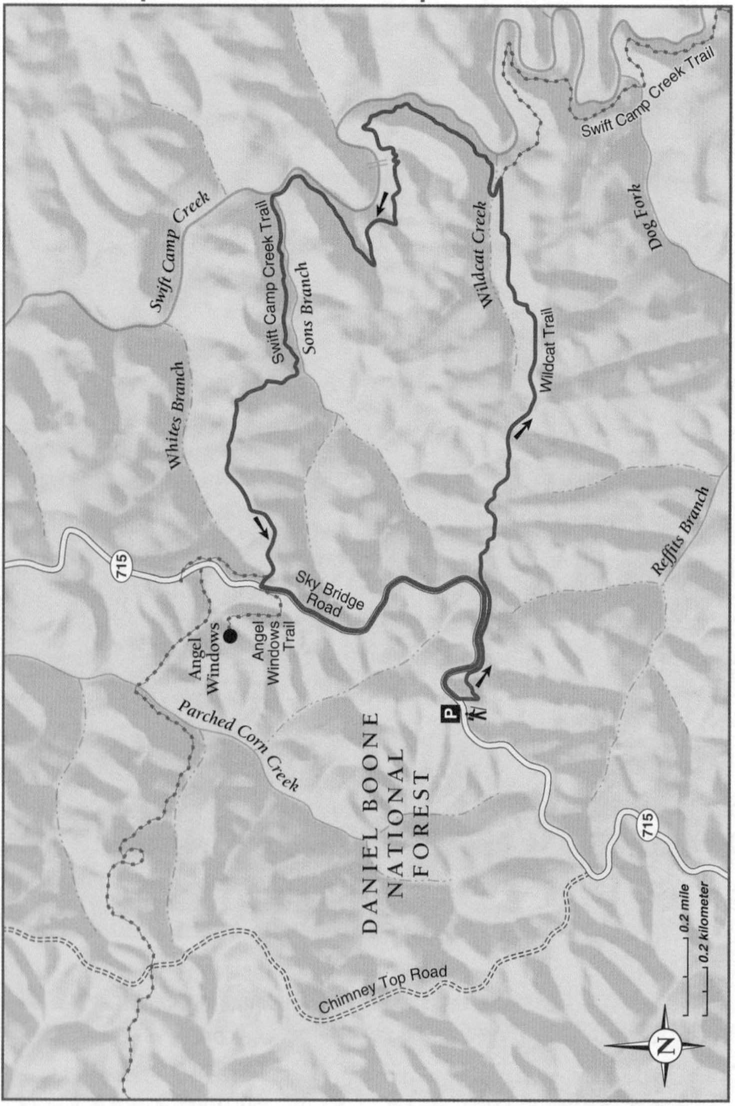

Swift Camp Creek Trail

Swift Camp Creek Trail

Swift Camp Creek

Swift Camp Creek Trail

Sons Branch

Whites Branch

Wildcat Creek

Wildcat Trail

Dog Fork

Reffits Branch

715

Sky Bridge Road

Angel Windows

Angel Windows Trail

Parched Corn Creek

P

DANIEL BOONE NATIONAL FOREST

715

Chimney Top Road

0.2 mile
0.2 kilometer

N

GPS TRAILHEAD COORDINATES: *Wildcat Trailhead* N37° 47.475' W83° 35.794'

DISTANCE & CONFIGURATION: 5.3-mile loop

HIGHLIGHTS: Rugged forest trails and creekside hiking

HIKING TIME: 3 hours

ELEVATION: 1,210' at the trailhead, descending to 754'

ACCESS: Open 24/7; vehicle pass required for overnight parking

MAPS: USGS *Pomeroyton;* USFS *Red River Gorge Geological Area*

FACILITIES: None

WHEELCHAIR ACCESS: None

COMMENTS: Dangerous cliffs are present and should be avoided, especially by children.

CONTACTS: Daniel Boone National Forest, Cumberland Ranger District, Gladie Cultural-Environmental Learning Center: 606-663-8100, tinyurl.com/gladie

Overview

Two trails create a quiet, seldom-used loop through the primitive Clifty Wilderness, descending to Swift Camp Creek and passing numerous cliff formations and water-cooled grottoes. The woods of this 12,600-acre wilderness, one of only two in Kentucky, are lush here, especially along the creek, where white-flowered rhododendrons lean out over the broad, slow Swift Camp Creek, and lichen blooms on the boulders scattered along the shores. Parts of the trail are in rough shape, having not been maintained adequately, but

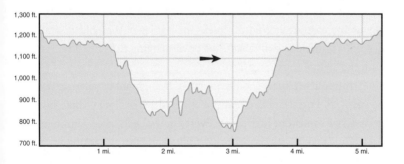

in other places the trail is broad and easy. The loop descends into the ravine of Wildcat Creek, which slips nearly invisibly through a wooded ravine to its confluence with Swift Camp Creek. The trail climbs for a distance away from the creek and finally returns to the water's edge along a series of sandy beaches; it then crosses and follows Sons Branch back toward the road through an open oak and pine forest. The last leg of this hike is an easy amble along the tree-shaded paved road back to Wildcat Trailhead.

Route Details

Beginning at the Wildcat Trailhead lot, cross the road to pick up the trail. In a short 0.1 mile, follow the sign for the Wildcat Trail to the left and continue east another 0.4 mile. The trail here, though new, can be overgrown and confusing. When you reach an old road, make a right. This is the original trail, which was rerouted recently. Once you're on the road, the trail immediately forks. To the right and up a short rise is a small but immaculately maintained cemetery. Continue on the Wildcat Trail to the left, heading east.

Much of the Wildcat Trail can be overgrown and unmaintained, and this can cause some anxiety. Follow the white diamond blazes into the forest. The trail will soon follow the ravine of Wildcat Creek, which is far below on the left. The Wildcat Trail traverses this forest 1.2 miles into the densely timbered Clifty Wilderness and eventually within earshot of Wildcat Creek. The last leg of the Wildcat Trail descends numerous switchbacks past overhanging cliffs to a junction with the Swift Camp Creek Trail.

Intrepid explorers should note that, though not detailed on the newest U.S. Forest Service map for the Red River Gorge, there is a decent-size sandstone arch across Swift Camp Creek called Timmons Arch. Only hikers with proper route-finding and bushwhacking skills should attempt to find it.

Swift Camp Creek Trail, like the Wildcat Trail, will also feel primitive and unmaintained. Expect to push lots of branches aside,

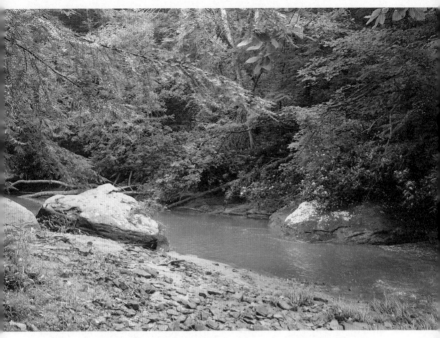

THIS BEACH ALONG SWIFT CAMP CREEK IS A GREAT PLACE TO TAKE A BREAK.

and watch your footing, especially on the section that follows the contours of Swift Camp Creek. Much of this trail will be loose rocks and muddy streams.

Go left on Swift Camp Creek Trail and quickly cross Wildcat Creek, where trilliums bloom in spring. Here the trail heads mostly north for a distance. Shortly after the Wildcat Creek crossing, watch for a couple of side trails leading to the right. These provide the first access to a beach along Swift Camp Creek. It is worth your time to see the wide, slow creek. With a number of boulders, sandy beaches, and rhododendron tangles, this makes a good rest spot. It will also be the last access point for some time, as the majority of the Swift Camp Creek Trail follows the creek from high above the water.

After the beach, the route climbs out of the ravine, staying high above it for the next 1.3 miles. The path climbs steadily, crossing several seasonal streams. It also passes a number of grottoes, one with a small waterfall sliding over an overhanging cliff. On a hot day, the air is noticeably cooler here, which makes it a good place to catch your breath. Watch (and listen) for frogs.

The trail returns to the creek at the 3-mile mark. From there, the hike follows the water for only 0.25 mile, but it is a lovely and cool 0.25 mile, especially in summer heat. You'll find opportunities to rest along this stretch of creek as well. The trail soon arrives at Sons Branch, a feeder creek descending noisily through massive boulders. Ford this small creek and go immediately left (west) up a rock stairway.

The trail quickly begins the long ascent away from Swift Camp Creek, following Sons Branch in a wooded ravine to the left. Continue on Swift Camp Creek Trail for 1 mile through increasingly open woods and watch for an unmarked junction; the trail to the right is the official Swift Camp Creek Trail, which leads to its upper trailhead on KY 715. To shorten the loop, go left instead along an exposed rock shelf. This unofficial side trail also reaches KY 715, but across from the Angel Windows Trailhead lot. Go left on the road and follow it 1.1 miles back to the Wildcat Trailhead lot on the right.

Directions

From Exit 40 off Bert T. Combs Mountain Parkway, go right on KY 15/ KY 715 for 1 mile, then follow KY 715 right for 3 miles to the Wildcat Trailhead parking area on the left. The trail begins just across the road.

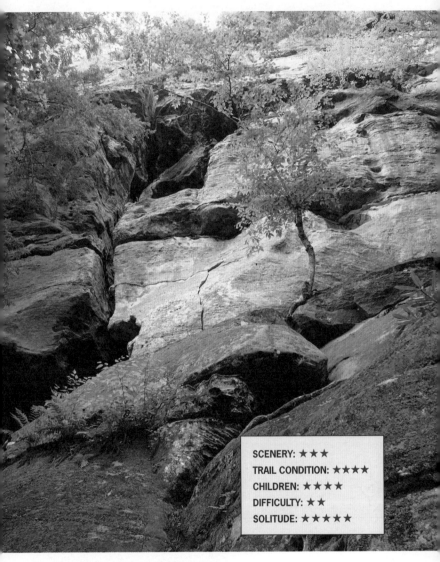

SCENERY: ★★★
TRAIL CONDITION: ★★★★
CHILDREN: ★★★★
DIFFICULTY: ★★
SOLITUDE: ★★★★★

ROCK-CLIMBING AREA ON TOWER ROCK

Tower Rock

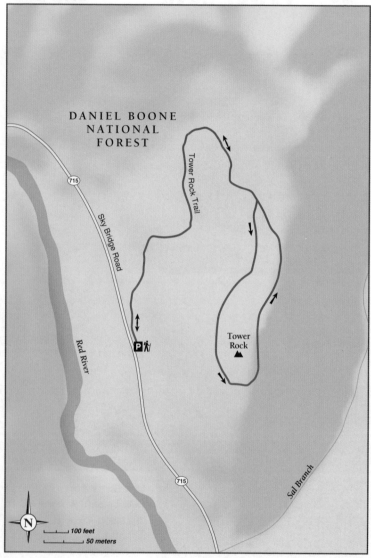

GPS TRAILHEAD COORDINATES: *Tower Rock Trailhead* N37° 49.706' W83° 35.921'

DISTANCE & CONFIGURATION: 1-mile balloon

HIGHLIGHTS: A monolithic rock formation popular with rock climbers

HIKING TIME: 1 hour

ELEVATION: 721' at the trailhead, ascending to 998'

ACCESS: Open 24/7; vehicle pass required for overnight parking

MAPS: USGS *Pomeroyton;* USFS *Red River Gorge Geological Area*

FACILITIES: None

WHEELCHAIR ACCESS: None

COMMENTS: Dangerous cliffs are present and should be avoided, especially by children.

CONTACTS: Daniel Boone National Forest, Cumberland Ranger District, Gladie Cultural-Environmental Learning Center: 606-663-8100, tinyurl.com/gladie

Overview

Hulking and hidden above the Red River is the monolithic Tower Rock, known to rock climbers but virtually unknown to hikers, and even then there may be no one there at all. The trailhead is virtually unmarked but for a small trail sign along the road. Even the parking area is obscure. That said, this is a short and pleasant hike into the edge of the Clifty Wilderness, through rhododendron thickets and tall hardwoods, to a sandstone cathedral rising 90 feet above the forest floor. The climb to Tower Rock is easy and makes a good hike for kids.

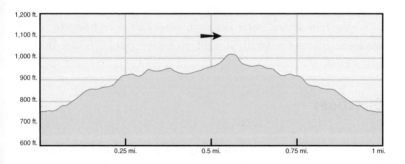

Route Details

The limited parking spots for this trail lie on the Red River (south) side of KY 715 in the thin gravel pullouts. From those spots, cross the road to the almost unnoticeable sign for Tower Rock Trail 229. The trail heads in a northeasterly direction and climbs gradually into the forest of rhododendrons and tall hardwoods, an easy stroll. Nearing the rock, the trail curves around to the south. At 0.4 mile you'll reach the northern end of Tower Rock, a 90-foot-high tower of sandstone conglomerate. The rock here cannot be climbed except on a rope, so do not attempt to do so. You will, however, notice the bolts fixed to the smooth walls in several places.

From here, the trail loops around the rock, though the path is poorly marked. The return trail on the left is obscured, so it's easiest to go straight, following the scant white diamonds on the trees. At one point, the trail goes through the crack of a split boulder. Simply keep Tower Rock on your left, following this primitive trail around the base of Tower Rock 0.2 mile, and it is extremely unlikely that you'll get lost. The trail passes rock climbing walls and old-growth pines, and it is a good idea to stop occasionally and simply look up. This is the only real view you will get of Tower Rock; nowhere along this trail or even the road can you see the tower in its entirety. The reward of this hike, though, and especially for kids, is to explore the base of Tower Rock, which is impressive in its own right.

The trail circles Tower Rock counterclockwise and returns to the more obvious main trail. Go right, descending gradually to return to the road.

Directions

From Exit 40 off Bert T. Combs Mountain Parkway, go right on KY 15/KY 715 for 1 mile, then follow KY 715 right for 8.7 miles to the Tower Rock Trail. Watch for a few pullout spots on the left. The trail begins just across the road.

Turtle Back Arch

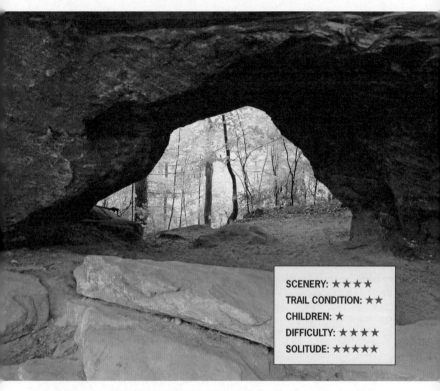

SCENERY: ★ ★ ★ ★
TRAIL CONDITION: ★ ★
CHILDREN: ★
DIFFICULTY: ★ ★ ★ ★
SOLITUDE: ★ ★ ★ ★

AN UNMARKED PATH TO TURTLE BACK ARCH ENSURES SOLITUDE ON THIS HIKE.

GPS TRAILHEAD COORDINATES:
Rock Bridge Recreation Area Trailhead N37° 46.211' W83° 33.978'

DISTANCE & CONFIGURATION: 4-mile loop

HIGHLIGHTS: Rugged forest trails, creekside hiking, and an off-trail adventure to visit Turtle Back Arch

HIKING TIME: 3 hours

ELEVATION: 1,178' at the arch; 886' along the creek

ACCESS: Open 24/7; vehicle pass required for overnight parking

MAPS: USGS *Pomeroyton;* USFS *Red River Gorge Geological Area*

FACILITIES: Restrooms at Rock Bridge Recreation Area

Turtle Back Arch

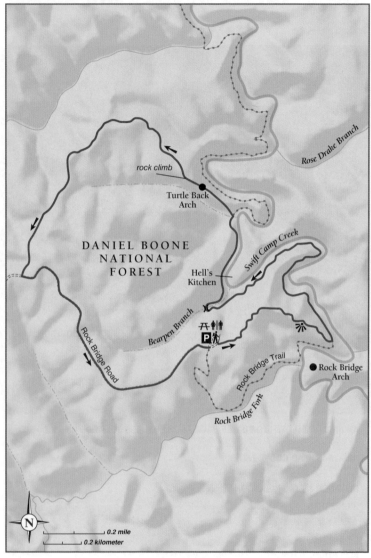

WHEELCHAIR ACCESS: None

COMMENTS: This trail requires route-finding skills, some bushwhacking, and a map and compass. Parts of this hike are on unmarked and unmaintained trails, and several cliff scrambles are required. Dangerous cliffs are present and should be avoided, especially by children. For a longer hike, combine this trip with the Rock Bridge Arch hike (Hike 9, page 68), adding only 0.9 mile to the walk.

CONTACTS: Daniel Boone National Forest, Cumberland Ranger District, Gladie Cultural-Environmental Learning Center: 606-663-8100, tinyurl.com/gladie

Overview

Of all the hikes in this book, this is the one that will take you a good distance from a maintained trail and into the Clifty Wilderness. Setting out from the popular Rock Bridge Recreation Area, the hike follows a paved path for a short distance before embarking on the wide and steady Swift Camp Creek Trail. The distance traveled along Swift Camp Creek follows a canyon known as Hell's Kitchen, hemmed in by sheer sandstone cliffs. To the west of the creek, up a trail so hidden it could well be missed, is Turtle Back Arch, set high on a ridge. A bit of off-trail bushwhacking leads past a good campsite and up the ridge to this small but interesting arch (actually, a double arch). From here, the going gets a bit rougher, so the faint of heart may want to claim victory and head back the way they came.

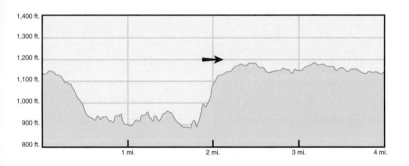

If, however, you can manage a bit of nontechnical climbing up a series of cliffs, you can continue on a loop along an old road that rides a high ridge over the wilderness. The abandoned road, though unmaintained for hiking, is easily discernible as it crosses a pine forest and returns to Rock Bridge Road. From there, the going is as easy as it gets, following the road back less than a mile to the picnic area and the end of the loop. Although you could conceivably bring kids, I discourage their climbing the cliffs and doing the loop. With endurance, they can make it up the easy, hillside pitch to the arch, but after that it's best for them to go back the way they came.

Route Details

From Rock Bridge Recreation Area, find the obvious restrooms. Just over the road from the restrooms is a signed trailhead, the beginning of the loop. Follow this mostly paved path downward, passing a good overlook on the right, and in only 0.5 mile you will arrive at the junction with Swift Camp Creek Trail. Turn left, following this well-beaten path north along the creek. A side trail early on this stretch goes down to the creek, where remnants of an old splash dam are a reminder of the logging days in this area. For most of the distance, though, the creek will be inaccessible.

Notice how quickly the creek disappears into a sandstone canyon; this is Hell's Kitchen. At the 1.2-mile mark, the trail crosses a footbridge over Bearpen Branch and follows what looks like the bottom of a creek, especially after rains. Soon after, Swift Camp Creek Trail passes between two large, obvious boulders. On the left a path leads to a rock shelter, the site of an old moonshine still. At 1.4 miles the trail crosses an unnamed stream with a waterfall on the right. Cross this stream and look immediately left for a path through a tunnel of rhododendrons. This is the way to Turtle Back Arch.

From here, route-finding skills will prove valuable, though the going is not too difficult. Head through the tunnel of rhodies and emerge at a large campsite. Note the trails leading away from it and going uphill. Follow the most obvious one about 300 feet to the top of the ridge. From here, continue on this trail that leads to the west along the side of the ridge. In the course of about 200 feet, you will need to cross over two rock faces, the second about 15 feet in height, which requires a bit of climbing. This will take you to the top of a ridge. At the ridgetop, continue west to another pronounced rock face, going to the left of the face until you reach the obvious opening of the arch (N37° 46.648' W83° 34.025').

This is a good place to stop and rest. For kids, this is also an optimal time to turn back. If you choose to continue on the loop, the remainder of the hike will be a small adventure. Go under the arch and turn right (here you will see Turtle Back's smaller arch), following the rock face to its end. At the edge of the rock face, circle it until you find the safest place to ascend (which, for me, was around on the edge and a bit farther along the opposite side, where some trees provided handholds). Once on top of this ridge, walk to the west, as if you were doubling back toward Turtle Back Arch. At a second, very obvious and tall rock face, go to the left side of it. You will see a climbing route up the sandstone with some roots and small tree trunks to use for leverage. At the top of this climb, follow a faint trail to the left (west).

From here, the hike grows easier as you follow this path along the ridge and through the forest until, at 2.1 miles, it dead-ends on an old road. Turn left, following this old road an easy 0.6 mile to gravel Rock Bridge Road. Once on the road, go left (east), walking the easy 0.9 mile back to the picnic area and your vehicle.

Directions

Take Exit 40 off Bert T. Combs Mountain Parkway. At the stop sign, go right on KY 15/KY 715 for 1 mile. Where the roads split in the small community of Pine Ridge, go right on KY 715 1 mile north, turning right onto gravel Rock Bridge Road (Forest Service Road 24). Continue 3 miles to the road's end and the parking area, at Rock Bridge Recreation Area.

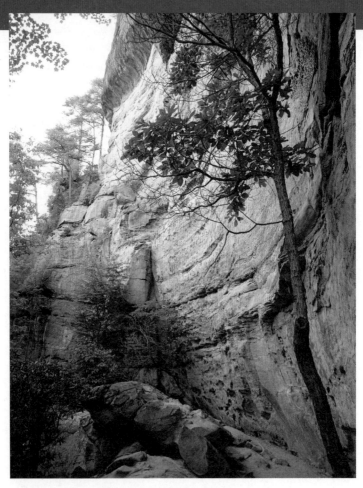

CLIFFS ALONG THE SHELTOWEE TRACE *(Hike 22, page 137)*

22 BALANCED ROCK AND ROCK GARDEN TRAIL 137

23 HENSON'S CAVE ARCH 142

24 HOOD'S BRANCH–SAND GAP LOOP 147

25 THE ORIGINAL TRAIL 153

Balanced Rock and Rock Garden Trail

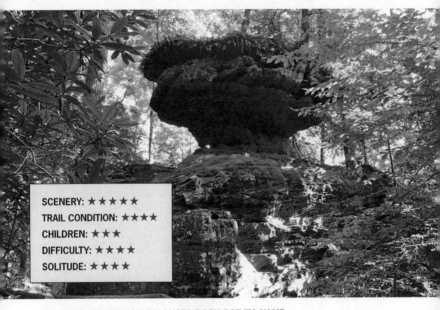

SCENERY: ★★★★★
TRAIL CONDITION: ★★★★
CHILDREN: ★★★
DIFFICULTY: ★★★★
SOLITUDE: ★★★★

IT'S CLEAR TO SEE HOW BALANCED ROCK GOT ITS NAME.

GPS TRAILHEAD COORDINATES: *Hemlock Lodge parking lot*
N37° 46.585' W83° 40.858'

DISTANCE & CONFIGURATION: 2.5-mile loop

HIGHLIGHTS: Natural Bridge, one of Kentucky's most famous arches, and stunning viewpoints

HIKING TIME: 2 hours

ELEVATION: 850' at trailhead, ascending to 1,333'

ACCESS: Day use only; no overnight camping allowed. Hikers must be off the trail by sunset. No dogs are allowed on trails in Natural Bridge State Resort Park.

MAPS: USGS *Slade;* Natural Bridge State Resort Park Trail Guide

FACILITIES: Restrooms in Hemlock Lodge and shelters along the Original Trail

WHEELCHAIR ACCESS: None

COMMENTS: Dangerous cliffs are present and should be avoided, especially by children.

CONTACTS: Natural Bridge State Resort Park: 606-663-2214 or 800-325-1710, parks.ky.gov/parks/resortparks/natural-bridge

Balanced Rock and Rock Garden Trail

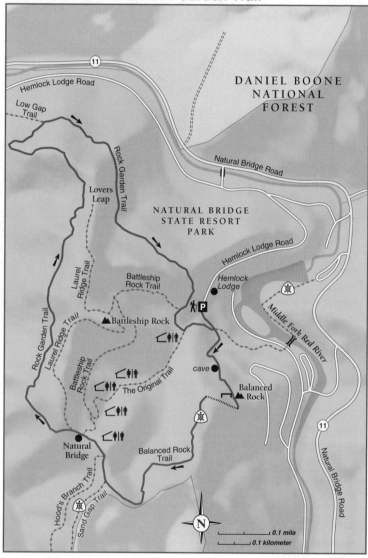

DANIEL BOONE NATIONAL FOREST

NATURAL BRIDGE STATE RESORT PARK

Hemlock Lodge Road

Natural Bridge Road

Low Gap Trail

Hemlock Lodge Road

Lovers Leap

Rock Garden Trail

Laurel Ridge Trail

Battleship Rock Trail

Hemlock Lodge

Middle Fork Red River

Battleship Rock

Battleship Rock Trail

The Original Trail

cave

Balanced Rock

Rock Garden Trail

Laurel Ridge Trail

Natural Bridge

Balanced Rock Trail

Hood's Branch Trail

Sand Gap Trail

Natural Bridge Road

N

0.1 mile
0.1 kilometer

Overview

Naturally, anyone visiting Natural Bridge State Resort Park is going to visit the namesake of the park, the soaring sandstone arch rising above the forest. Chances are that if they are tourists, they will climb to see the sights via the Original Trail, arguably the most popular trail in the entire state of Kentucky. But there are other ways to get to Natural Bridge. Balanced Rock Trail is one of those ways, and it will quickly weed out the unambitious. Following the route of the famous Sheltowee Trace, this trail literally climbs, via what seems like a continuous stone stairway, nearly 500 feet in just over 0.5 mile. The reward is that you'll not only miss the crowds but also get to see some truly humbling cliffs and rock formations, including the precarious Balanced Rock. In fact, this hike is all about rock. Once you reach Natural Bridge, you can take any number of trails back, but this hike continues to tour the rock formations via the Rock Garden Trail, which traces its way around Laurel Ridge, Lovers Leap, and Lookout Point, ultimately joining the Battleship Rock Trail and reconnecting with the Original Trail. The mileage seems easy, but this hike is challenging. It's also fun.

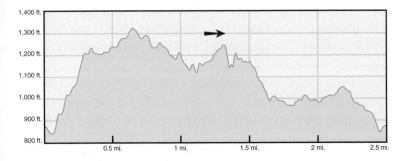

Route Details

From the signboard at the end of the Hemlock Lodge parking area, follow the paved path past the start of the Original Trail to the Balanced Rock Trail on the right. The limestone stairway you see is only the beginning of what will be nearly one continuous stairway. Set out on this trail, part of the Sheltowee Trace that crosses the Red River Gorge roughly north to south. At the top of the stairway, the trail turns sharply left and passes a large cave. (Were you allowed to do so, this cave could lead you through the cliff to its opposite end on the Original Trail; however, it is securely fenced off.)

The trail climbs again, up more steps and around a switchback. At 0.2 mile the trail passes Balanced Rock, which will be on the left. There is a bench here, and you'll likely be tempted to sit and ponder not only this solid-sandstone block but also the sheer limestone cliffs that rise around it. Chances are you'll need to rest up, for the remainder of this trail can be grueling.

The next 0.5 mile starts out with stairway after stairway, levels out for a short distance along a ridge with views, and then charges up the last 150 feet to the sandstone slopes leading to the arch. At the top of this ridge, you are within a short walk of Natural Bridge. Walk north through the pines, passing a trail junction on the left at 0.7 mile; here you leave the Sheltowee Trace, which veers off to the south toward the Daniel Boone National Forest, following the Sand Gap Trail through the outer edges of Natural Bridge State Resort Park. Continue straight to a large shelter. Just beyond is Natural Bridge. Stop atop the arch, but beware of the edges.

When you're ready to continue, follow a stairway down the southwest corner of the arch. Squeeze through the narrow gap known around here as Fat Man's Misery, and then emerge beneath the arch. Looking straight ahead, staying on the western side of the edge, you will intersect the Rock Garden Trail. Follow this picturesque trail north along the cliffs, taking note of the amazing rock formations in the cliffs, the rock pockmarked and smoothed through weathering.

This is also a great place to see the formations known as concretions, the swirling patterns in sandstone caused by the weathering of sandstone away from the more resistant iron oxides. The Rock Garden Trail follows the sides of Laurel Ridge for 1 mile and, after descending a tight stone stairway along a cliff, meets with the Low Gap Trail, which leads down 0.5 mile to the base of the sky lift. Stay to the right at this junction, heading east on Rock Garden Trail.

The trail is now better maintained, entering into a sunlit forest where it crosses another kind of rock garden. For a distance, the forest floor is strewn with enormous, house-size boulders sprouting everything from moss and ferns to trees. After 0.5 mile the Rock Garden Trail ends at Battleship Rock Trail. Go left on Battleship Rock Trail, following signs for Hemlock Lodge, and in about 400 feet you will emerge on the Original Trail. Go left and downhill, returning to the paved path and ending the loop. From here, simply go left and uphill on the paved path to return to the Hemlock Lodge lot.

Directions

From Exit 33 off Bert T. Combs Mountain Parkway, drive south on KY 11 for 2 miles to the main entrance of Natural Bridge State Resort Park. Turn right into the entrance, then take an immediate left, following signs for Hemlock Lodge 0.3 mile to the lot. Don't park beyond the lodge—those spaces are reserved for guests.

23 Henson's Cave Arch

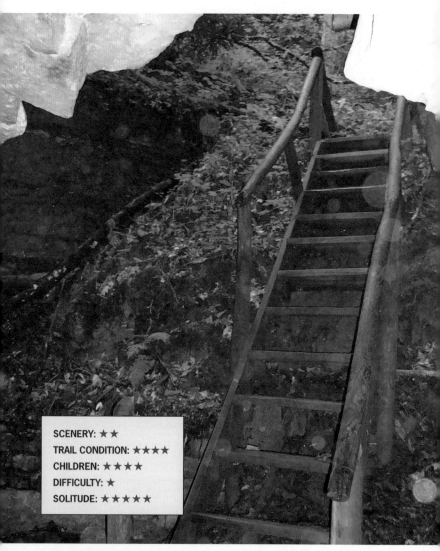

SCENERY: ★★
TRAIL CONDITION: ★★★★
CHILDREN: ★★★★
DIFFICULTY: ★
SOLITUDE: ★★★★★

FROM HENSON'S CAVE ARCH, A STAIRWAY LEADS DOWN INTO A SINKHOLE, WHERE HIKERS GAIN A DIFFERENT PERSPECTIVE OF THE ARCH.

GPS TRAILHEAD COORDINATES: *Whittleton Campground* N37° 46.811' W83° 40.492'

DISTANCE & CONFIGURATION: 0.8-mile out-and-back

HIGHLIGHTS: Forest walk and cave

HIKING TIME: 1 hour

ELEVATION: 764' at trailhead, with a gain of 240'

ACCESS: Day use only; no overnight camping on the trail allowed. Hikers must be off the trail by sunset. No dogs are allowed on trails in Natural Bridge State Resort Park.

MAPS: USGS *Slade;* Natural Bridge State Resort Park Trail Guide

FACILITIES: Restrooms in Whittleton Campground

WHEELCHAIR ACCESS: None

COMMENTS: Easy hike, especially for children, but take care near the cave.

CONTACTS: Natural Bridge State Resort Park: 606-663-2214 or 800-325-1710, parks.ky.gov/parks/resortparks/natural-bridge

Overview

If you're planning a trip to Natural Bridge State Resort Park, you should really think about staying for at least a night, or even two. There's so much to see that you couldn't possibly take it all in within the confines of a single day. Natural Bridge is a great place to camp, too, and the Whittleton Campground is absolutely lovely, although it can be difficult to find a spot there on crowded holiday weekends. Whittleton Branch flows through the campground on its way to the Middle Fork of the Red River, and several campsites lie along the creek. After a day of trekking, Whittleton Campground makes for a good respite. It's also home base for good hikes. One of the most famous trips, the 1.2-mile hike up Whittleton Fork to the Whittleton Arch, starts in the campground. But another, shorter, lesser-known hike starts here too: the trail to Henson's Cave Arch.

It's tough to say exactly what Henson's Cave Arch is. It's a limestone formation that is sort of an arch, sort of a cave, definitely a grotto, and, depending on the season, also a waterfall. This short (0.4-mile) trail makes a good evening stroll or an early-morning warm-up. It also can be a precursor to the nearby Whittleton Branch Trail as a bit of limbering up for an extended hike. Because of its ease and proximity to the campground, this is one of the few hikes in the

Henson's Cave Arch

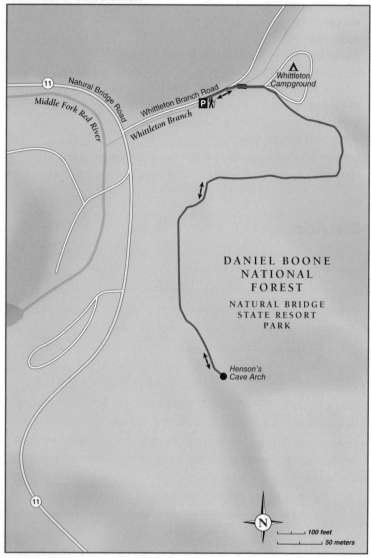

11

Natural Bridge Road

Whittleton Branch Road

Middle Fork Red River

Whittleton Branch

P

Whittleton
Campground

DANIEL BOONE
NATIONAL
FOREST

NATURAL BRIDGE
STATE RESORT
PARK

Henson's
Cave Arch

11

N

100 feet

50 meters

Red River Gorge that is quite safe for children, provided they keep back from the unprotected skylight hole that forms the "arch" and are careful on the stairs leading into the "cave."

Route Details

To begin the short hike to Henson's Cave Arch, start near the Whittleton Campground's main entrance. Just to the east of the check-in booth and a woodshed, along the creek, is a small parking area for day hikers. About 250 feet beyond the parking area, a footbridge and a roadway cross Whittleton Branch; cross the creek here, heading toward the bathhouse with the washer-dryer sets and drink machines. Walking 500 feet up this road, go toward campsite A7, set alongside a smaller creek. The Henson's Arch Trail begins at a well-marked trailhead by a large signboard.

Cross a footbridge over the small creek and head to the right up the trail. The first 0.1 mile climbs the hillside in a somewhat rugged fashion, gaining about 30 feet of elevation; this section has some loose rocks and can be slippery in wet weather. From here the trail levels and heads west, occasionally rising gently for another 0.2 mile. The path follows the hillside around and gradually turns to the south,

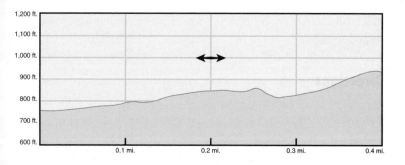

toward the traffic noise on KY 11. The maple-and-hemlock woods here, though, are mostly quiet and will be largely free of hikers.

At 0.3 mile the trail climbs toward a gap in a cliff. To the right and below you, the seasonal stream that carved this notch in the limestone will be flowing. The trail climbs about 140 feet over the final 0.1 mile through the gap, ending in a small valley. You will soon see the wooden guardrails around the arch.

Be careful when you approach this limestone arch formation in wet weather. The wooden guardrails narrow and lead to the stairway. Avoid the smaller hole directly on your right. The trail officially ends at this wooden stairway that can be quite slick when wet, and at any rate it is missing one of its rails. The stairway descends into the cave, which can also be described as a grotto. If it has been raining any-time recently, a waterfall will be dripping into this cave. Once you've reached the bottom, notice to the left that there is a small grotto and, at the top of that, a skylight hole; this is the "arch" referred to in the landmark's name. The bottom of these two chambers will likely be wet rock or standing water.

For a look at the skylight hole from above, climb back out and walk around the larger hole. Note that this skylight hole, as well as the rest of the area around the stairwell entrance, is unprotected, which is to say that there are no guardrails. Above the cave, the small creek stretches back into the small valley, though there is no official trail in that direction. It's best to end the hike here and return the way you came.

Directions

From Exit 33 off Bert T. Combs Mountain Parkway, drive south on KY 11 for 2.2 miles to the entrance of Whittleton Campground. Turn left into the campground and park on the right in a small lot just beyond the woodshed. Follow the road into the campground and turn right, over a bridge. The trail begins near campsite A7.

Hood's Branch–
Sand Gap Loop

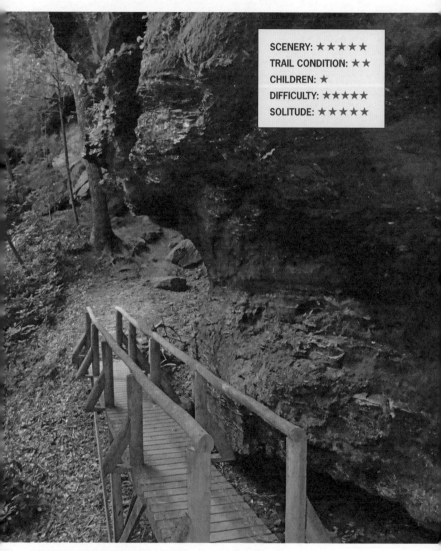

SCENERY: ★ ★ ★ ★ ★
TRAIL CONDITION: ★ ★
CHILDREN: ★
DIFFICULTY: ★ ★ ★ ★ ★
SOLITUDE: ★ ★ ★ ★ ★

ONE OF TWO FOOTBRIDGES ON THE HOOD'S BRANCH TRAIL THAT CROSSES A
SWAMPY SECTION

Hood's Branch–Sand Gap Loop

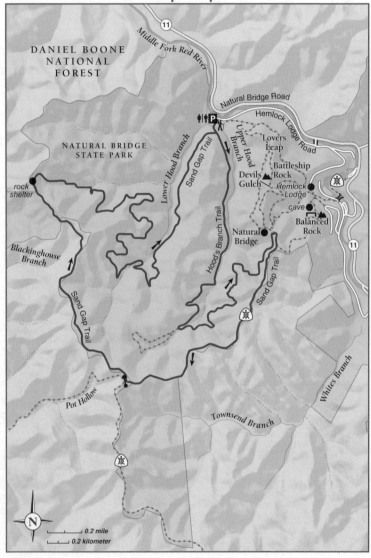

GPS TRAILHEAD COORDINATES: N37° 46.895' W83° 41.470'

DISTANCE & CONFIGURATION: 10.5-mile loop

HIGHLIGHTS: Natural Bridge, one of Kentucky's most famous arches, and stunning viewpoints

HIKING TIME: 6 hours

ELEVATION: 747' at trailhead, ascending to 1,297'

ACCESS: Day use only; no overnight camping allowed. Hikers must be off the trail by sunset. No dogs are allowed on trails in Natural Bridge State Resort Park.

MAPS: USGS *Slade;* Natural Bridge State Resort Park Trail Guide

FACILITIES: Restrooms at the trailhead and one shelter along Hood's Branch Trail

WHEELCHAIR ACCESS: None

COMMENTS: Dangerous cliffs are present and should be avoided, especially by children. This is a long, virtually unmaintained, very difficult trail. Water sources are few, depending on the season. Give yourself plenty of time to do this hike: at least 5–6 hours.

CONTACTS: Natural Bridge State Resort Park: 606-663-2214 or 800-325-1710, parks.ky.gov/parks/resortparks/natural-bridge

Overview

Of all the hikes in Natural Bridge State Resort Park—in fact, of all the hikes in the entire Red River Gorge area—this one is without a doubt one of the most demanding and difficult. You have several options for climbing to and descending from Natural Bridge, but this route is the longest. Because of the difficulty, expect extreme solitude here. You

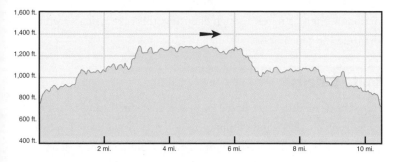

should also expect to occasionally get anxious over trail junctions, thick rhododendron thickets, and endless numbers of spiderwebs strung across the trail. On the other hand, because of the relative lack of human visitors, you can also expect to see wildlife: wild turkeys roosting in the trees, deer in the thickets, or snakes along the trail. Be cautious, come prepared, and bring ample food and water. Because of the physical demands of this hike, you'll need fluids and energy.

Hood's Branch Trail is the initial ascent, following Upper Hood Branch through its ravine to the extreme headwaters of this creek. The trail climbs steadily and just as suddenly emerges beneath the massive span of Natural Bridge. Greenery abounds along this portion of the hike, and the first leg is the easiest. The second leg, however, can be punishing. Sand Gap Trail follows a 2-mile stretch of the Sheltowee Trace along the boundary of the state park, following a long ridge on what was once a logging road. Don't let the ease fool you; once this stretch of trail veers off from the Sheltowee, it begins a long, tiring, and meandering journey through the backcountry, tripping along vista-lined ridges, descending through overgrown woods, passing rock shelters, and finally following the Lower Hood's Branch back to the trailhead, along stretches populated with nettles and poison ivy. A bit of good news: this loop actually traverses a nature preserve, which affords protection to the rock formations along this route. Though daunting, this hike is doable with fortitude and preparation.

Route Details

From the trailhead, start uphill on a set of deteriorating wooden steps, switchbacking and climbing to a junction within 0.1 mile. This will be the end of the loop; for now, go left, following Hood's Branch Trail. From here the path levels out, following the west bank of Upper Hood Branch. At 0.6 mile a wooden shelter built by the Civilian Conservation Corps in the 1930s sits on a rise to the right.

The trail crosses the creek and boggy areas several times on wooden bridges, and the forest gets increasingly deeper.

At 1.5 miles the trail reaches a junction with another trail on the right. This is the short (0.75-mile) Upper Hood's Branch Loop. Continue to the left, crossing the creek on a small bridge. At nearly the 2-mile mark, you will make the last creek crossing before making the final climb. The trail passes cliffs and a rock shelter, and then pitches steeply to the 3-mile mark and the base of Natural Bridge. Go directly to the right, through the narrow fracture and up the stairway to the top of the arch. If you wish to consider the view, go to the left and be careful near the edge. Otherwise, head to the right along the exposed sandstone slopes. This short stretch is the top end of the Balanced Rock Trail; follow it 0.1 mile to a junction.

The junction is clearly signed as the Sand Gap Trail. The entire trail before you constitutes the Sheltowee Trace, which traverses nearly 20 miles of the Red River Gorge area. To the left, the Sheltowee descends the Balanced Rock Trail to the main part of the park. This hike goes to the right, following the Sand Gap Trail. Note the sign that insists you give yourself 5–6 hours to complete this trail. The trail will be blazed with white diamonds and the white turtle symbol.

The next 1.6 miles follow a ridge along a former logging road. The going is easy, and the trail quickly enters Natural Bridge State Nature Preserve. At the 4.6-mile mark, you'll come upon a confusing junction: the trail appears to go straight ahead to a gate, but this is not part of the loop. The Sheltowee Trace indeed goes straight through this gate, continuing south toward the Kentucky River and Daniel Boone National Forest. Instead, watch closely to the right for a sharp turn before the gate (some of the national forest signs are overgrown here, but there is a large wooden state-park sign, only easily seen if you're coming from the opposite direction).

After you turn right, the next 0.4 mile remains fairly level and easy, following the old road through a forest of predominantly high-elevation oaks and pines. For the most part, the trail remains clear as it crosses the ridgetop and eventually moves away from it; continue to keep an eye out for blazes. At the far end of the ridgetop, about the 6.5-mile mark, the trail begins to descend a bit into the woods, heading north. As it arcs around and heads south, a decent-size shallow cave appears on the cliff to the left. From here, the trail descends into the headwaters of Lower Hood Branch and zigzags like mad, crossing creek after creek, roller-coastering along ravines and through overgrown rhododendron thickets. This is by far the most tiring part of the hike. At 8.7 miles the trail begins to settle into a level rhythm along the gully of Lower Hood Branch. You'll cross a few bridges and pass a few benches, and at 10 miles the trail leaves the nature preserve. In 0.4 mile the trail ends at the Hood's Branch Trail, ending the loop. Turn left and descend the final 0.1 mile back to the minigolf course and the parking lot.

Directions

From Exit 33 off Bert T. Mountain Parkway, drive south on KY 11 for 2 miles to the main entrance of Natural Bridge State Resort Park. Turn right into the entrance, and then take an immediate right, following the road 0.7 mile to a large parking area on the left, by a minigolf course. The trail begins at the edge of the woods, behind the course.

25 The Original Trail

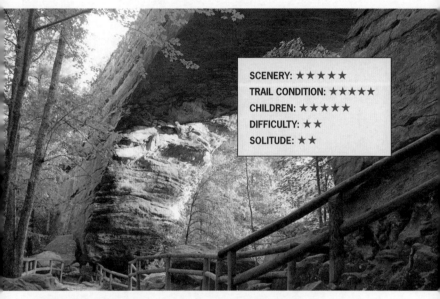

SCENERY: ★ ★ ★ ★ ★
TRAIL CONDITION: ★ ★ ★ ★ ★
CHILDREN: ★ ★ ★ ★ ★
DIFFICULTY: ★ ★
SOLITUDE: ★ ★

A TRAIL BUILT IN THE 1890s BY A RAILROAD COMPANY LEADS TO THE PARK'S NAMESAKE.

GPS TRAILHEAD COORDINATES: *Hemlock Lodge parking lot*
N37° 46.585' W83° 40.858'

DISTANCE & CONFIGURATION: 2.8-mile balloon

HIGHLIGHTS: Natural Bridge, one of Kentucky's most famous arches, and stunning viewpoints

HIKING TIME: 2 hours

ELEVATION: 850' at the trailhead, ascending to 1,333'

ACCESS: Day use only; no overnight camping allowed. Hikers must be off the trail by sunset. No dogs are allowed on trails in Natural Bridge State Resort Park.

MAPS: USGS *Slade;* Natural Bridge State Resort Park Trail Guide

FACILITIES: Restrooms in Hemlock Lodge and shelters along the Original Trail

WHEELCHAIR ACCESS: None

COMMENTS: Dangerous cliffs are present and should be avoided, especially by children.

CONTACTS: Natural Bridge State Resort Park: 606-663-2214 or 800-325-1710, parks.ky.gov/parks/resortparks/natural-bridge

The Original Trail

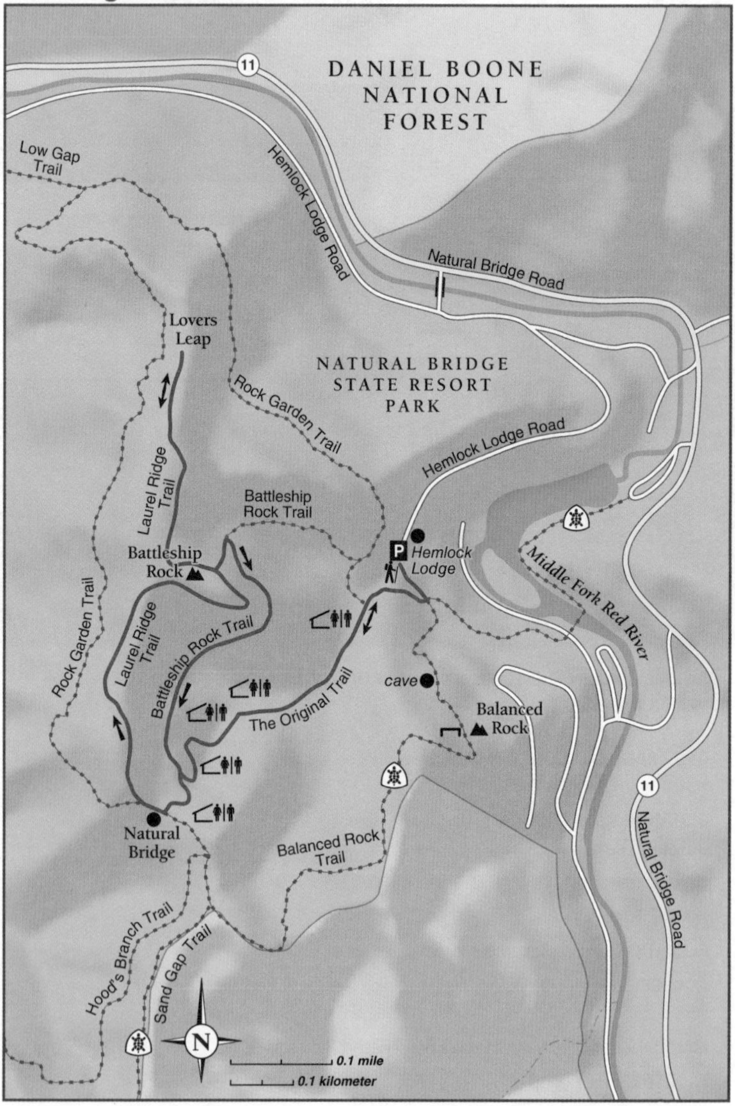

DANIEL BOONE
NATIONAL
FOREST

11

Low Gap
Trail

Hemlock Lodge Road

Natural Bridge Road

Lovers
Leap

NATURAL BRIDGE
STATE RESORT
PARK

Rock Garden Trail

Laurel Ridge Trail

Battleship
Rock Trail

Hemlock Lodge Road

Battleship
Rock

P Hemlock
   Lodge

Middle Fork Red River

Rock Garden Trail

Laurel Ridge Trail

Battleship Rock Trail

The Original Trail

cave

Balanced
Rock

11

Natural Bridge Road

Natural
Bridge

Balanced Rock
Trail

Hood's Branch Trail

Sand Gap Trail

N

0.1 mile

0.1 kilometer

Overview

The Lexington and Eastern Railroad, which used the Red River Gorge for extensive logging, donated land to the Commonwealth of Kentucky that eventually became the absolute gem known as Natural Bridge State Resort Park. But to give credit where credit is due, the railroad company set aside this landscape around Natural Bridge, which, according to the best sources, is the second-biggest arch (behind Grays Arch) in the Red River Gorge area. That said, Natural Bridge is the most popular arch and, hence, the most visited. The railroad company also built the Original Trail, easily one of the most heavily used 0.75-mile trails in the state. But don't let that fact sway you: Natural Bridge is a highlight of the Gorge, and if you avoid busy times, such as summer weekends, you can likely have Natural Bridge to yourself—at least for a while. But why stop at the arch, when the equally prominent Lookout Point lies just beyond? This tremendous overlook is where all the famous photos of Natural Bridge are taken. You can go farther, too, making an excellent short loop that also visits Lovers Leap and the Devil's Gulch. To create this loop, finish with the Battleship Rock Trail, which follows the amazing cliff formations beneath Laurel Ridge the whole way.

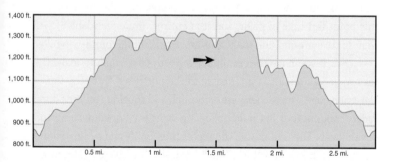

Route Details

From the parking area at Hemlock Lodge, walk past the lodge to the far lot. At a signboard, a paved path leads to the junction of trails, including the Original Trail.

The Original Trail heads uphill to the right. This wide, easy path makes for an enjoyable walk, but it's just steep enough to get your heart pumping a bit faster. Along the way, signboards detail the history of the area and describe the animals and mixed mesophytic forest through which the trail travels. You'll also be able to stop at one of several small shelters built by the Civilian Conservation Corps in the 1930s. The trail is so easy to distinguish that you'll have no trouble avoiding the other trails to the right, both of which are opposite ends of the looping Battleship Rock Trail. At 0.5 mile the Original Trail suddenly comes upon the soaring sandstone of Natural Bridge, largely shielded from view by the magnificent trees. Spend some time under the arch, the best place to view it. A number of trails fan out from the arch, including Battleship Rock, Rock Garden, and Hood's Branch Trails.

Walk under the arch. From the western side of the arch, look to the left (south). Here you will see the narrow notch known, perhaps crudely, as Fat Man's Misery. Walk through this notch, which brings you to a stone stairway up the side of the arch. At the top, go to the left and walk onto Natural Bridge. Stay away from the edges! There is no fencing, and the drop is pernicious and possibly deadly. To get to this point is a hike in itself, and it is entirely understandable if you wish to turn around and make this an easy 1.5-mile round-trip hike.

But if you have the stamina, it's worth your while to make the easy walk to Lookout Point, visible to the northeast from the top of Natural Bridge. To get there, cross the arch and continue on the Laurel Ridge Trail another 0.4 mile, following signs for Lookout Point and Lovers Leap. The trail passes the top of the sky lift and heads around the base of Battleship Rock. Soon after, you'll arrive at an obvious opening to the right—a wide, flat sandstone vista set on the edge of a precipitous cliff with tremendous views both over the surrounding Gorge area and, of course, the Natural Bridge. You could also turn around here and go back the way you came, but it's worth it to continue onward to Lovers Leap.

Continue north on the Laurel Ridge Trail, along the ridge. The trail passes two other spur trails along the way: Devil's Gulch and Needle's Eye, both steep stairways down to the Battleship Rock Trail. In another 0.2 mile the trail ends at Lovers Leap, which yields a view over the Middle Fork of the Red River and beyond. Be careful of the cliffs here. As long as you've come this far out, it's worth it to return not by the way you came but from below the cliffs.

Double back on the trail and head south about 0.1 mile. Though you could take either stairway down, Devil's Gulch Trail is the more adequately signed. Turn left onto Devil's Gulch Trail, quickly descending a steep, wooden staircase through a narrow, cliff-edged ravine. At the end of this trail, about 0.1 mile, you'll connect with Battleship Rock Trail. From here, it's most interesting to go right, following the base of the cliffs, passing great rock faces and formations, back to Natural Bridge and the Original Trail. Follow Battleship Rock Trail 0.5 mile to a junction. Either trail, left or right, will lead to the Original Trail, though if you want to take in Natural Bridge one last time, go to the right and uphill a short distance to the arch's base. Otherwise, veer left on the last leg of the Battleship Rock Trail to reconnect to the Original Trail, ending the loop portion of the hike. Go left on the Original Trail to return to the trailhead, only 0.75 mile away.

Directions

From Exit 33 off Bert T. Combs Mountain Parkway, drive south on KY 11 for 2 miles to the main entrance of Natural Bridge State Resort Park. Turn right into the entrance, and then take an immediate left, following signs for Hemlock Lodge 0.3 mile to the lot. Don't park beyond the lodge—those spaces are reserved for guests.

MORE TRAILS IN THE RED RIVER GORGE AREA

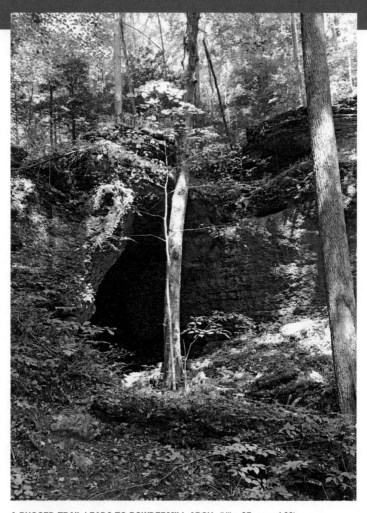

A RUGGED TRAIL LEADS TO POWDERMILL ARCH. *(Hike 27, page 163)*

26 PILOT KNOB STATE NATURE PRESERVE 159

27 POWDERMILL BRANCH TRAIL 163

28 WHITE'S BRANCH ARCH 168

Pilot Knob State Nature Preserve

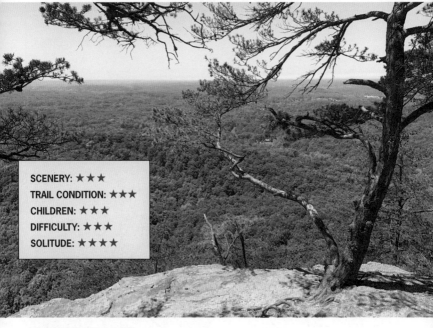

SCENERY: ★ ★ ★
TRAIL CONDITION: ★ ★ ★
CHILDREN: ★ ★ ★
DIFFICULTY: ★ ★ ★
SOLITUDE: ★ ★ ★ ★

VIEW FROM PILOT KNOB

GPS TRAILHEAD COORDINATES: *Pilot Knob Trailhead* N37° 54.723' W83° 56.697'

DISTANCE & CONFIGURATION: 4.5-mile loop

HIGHLIGHTS: Wooded terrain and a view over the Cumberland Plateau

HIKING TIME: 3 hours

ELEVATION: 800' at the trailhead, ascending to 1,420'

ACCESS: Open 24/7; vehicle pass required for overnight parking

MAPS: USGS *Levee*; trail map available online at eec.ky.gov/Nature-Preserves/Brochures /PilotKnobBrochure_color.pdf

FACILITIES: None

WHEELCHAIR ACCESS: None

COMMENTS: Dangerous cliffs are present and should be avoided, especially by children.

CONTACTS: Kentucky State Nature Preserves Commission: 502-782-7839, eec.ky.gov/Nature-Preserves/Locations/Pages/Pilot-Knob.aspx

Pilot Knob State Nature Preserve

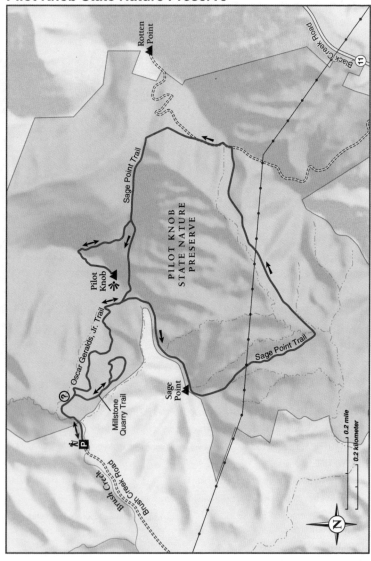

Overview

Just off the Bert T. Combs Mountain Parkway, west of Red River Gorge, lies the 742-acre Pilot Knob State Nature Preserve. Pieced together beginning with an original purchase made with The Nature Conservancy, the preserve covers creek bottoms, wooded ridges, and the highlight, a 730-foot-high sandstone outcrop that is said to have been visited by Daniel Boone and overlooks both the Bluegrass region and the beginning of the Cumberland Plateau. Though you can take a fairly steep incline straight to the top, it's worth it to tour the entire area, rich in wildflowers and native Kentucky hardwoods.

Route Details

From the parking lot, set out east on the trail, crossing Brush Creek. In 0.2 mile you'll reach the first junction; to the right is the 0.4-mile loop of the Millstone Quarry Trail, which is worth an exploration. To the left is the Oscar Geralds, Jr. Trail, which charges upward in just under a mile to the peak of Pilot Knob; to do so, simply continue upward, staying left at both junctions with the Sage Point Trail.

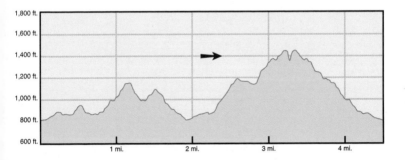

While this is a decent hike, though short, it's more challenging—and ultimately more fulfilling—to do the entire loop of the area. For the full loop, go right at the first junction with the Sage Point Trail. From here, you'll amble along ridgelines thick with oaks and hickories, dropping to another creek and wildflower-filled bottomland (sometimes crossing power line roads) and climbing again toward the prominence of Pilot Knob. After completing the 2-mile Sage Point Trail, watch for a trail to the right and follow it 0.4 mile to some stunning rock formations and, finally, the cliff-edge view that, in spring, flowers with mountain azalea.

To return, follow this trail back 0.4 mile, then turn right on the Oscar Geralds, Jr. Trail and follow it for 0.3 mile. As you descend, look up and to the right to see the cliff you were just on. Keep right at the junction with the Sage Point Trail, and again keep right after another 0.3 mile at the junction with the Millstone Quarry Trail. Return the last 0.25 mile to your car.

Directions

From Exit 16 off Bert T. Combs Mountain Parkway, go right (north) on KY 15 for 2.9 miles. Turn right on Brush Creek Road and follow it 1.6 miles to the parking lot at the end of the road. The trail begins at the edge of the lot.

27 Powdermill Branch Trail

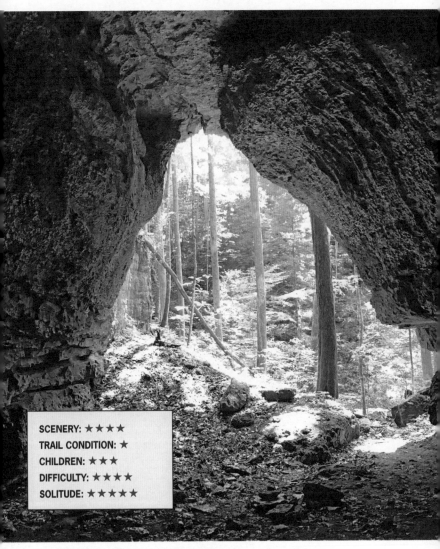

SCENERY: ★ ★ ★ ★
TRAIL CONDITION: ★
CHILDREN: ★ ★ ★
DIFFICULTY: ★ ★ ★ ★
SOLITUDE: ★ ★ ★ ★ ★

UNLIKE MANY ARCHES IN THE AREA, POWDERMILL ARCH CONSISTS OF
LIMESTONE, NOT SANDSTONE.

Powdermill Branch Trail

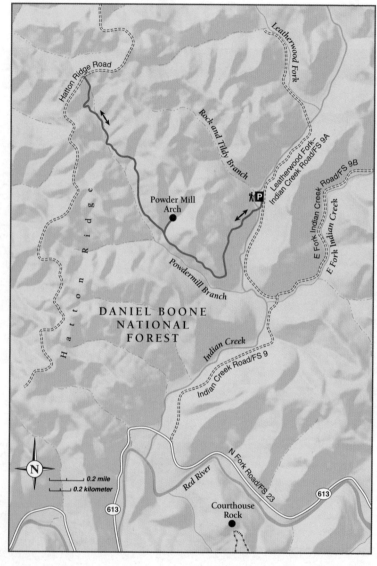

GPS TRAILHEAD COORDINATES: *Powdermill Branch Trailhead*
N37° 52.132' W83° 40.538'

DISTANCE & CONFIGURATION: 5-mile out-and-back

HIGHLIGHTS: Dense woods, a hidden arch, sinkholes, and a wooded ridgeline

HIKING TIME: 4.5 hours

ELEVATION: 625' at the trailhead, with an elevation gain of 665'

ACCESS: Open 24/7; vehicle pass required for overnight parking

MAPS: USGS *Slade;* USFS *Red River Gorge Geological Area*

FACILITIES: None

WHEELCHAIR ACCESS: None

COMMENTS: By summer, this trail is heavily overgrown. At this time, it is not actively maintained by the U.S. Forest Service. This trail is also open to mountain bikes and equestrians.

CONTACTS: Daniel Boone National Forest, Cumberland Ranger District, Gladie Cultural-Environmental Learning Center: 606-663-8100, tinyurl.com/gladie

Overview

I decided, in the course of researching this book, to include the Powdermill Trail, a relatively unknown, and frankly quite rugged, trail. To my knowledge, it's not heavily hiked; in fact, the trail gets crowded with poison ivy, greenbrier, and a number of weeds happy to stick to your socks. It's not even within the Red River Gorge Geological Area. So why include it at all? Because I found this to be one of the most

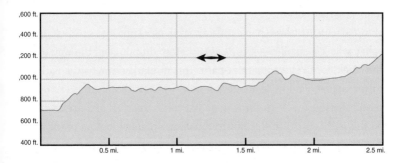

rewarding trails in the whole area. During one hike, I saw absolutely no one else—so there's a good chance for solitude. The quiet is pervasive, save the wind in the trees on Hatton Ridge, the trail's terminus, and the occasional sound of Powdermill Branch, which for the most part is inaccessible from the trail. Plus, there are a couple of geological wonders here: the impressive Powdermill Arch, the smaller Wolf Pen Arch, and a number of substantial sinkholes. My advice is simple: wear long pants, spray yourself thoroughly with bug spray, and watch for birds—I saw an ovenbird on this trail, a kind of warbler. The trail is apparent, though faint at times. I had no trouble finding my way, but be sure to bring a map and compass.

Route Details

From the signboard, the first small stretch of trail loops along the curve of Indian Creek—the beginning is obvious enough, though for a short distance you'll make your way through waist-high wildflowers before coming down to the creek bank itself, beside a campsite and beneath the road you drove in on.

There is no bridge, so you will have to ford the creek. If the water is low, you can rock-hop, and if not, you'll probably want to remove your boots. On the other side, take the trail headed into the woods, which soon climbs uphill to the right before leveling off and following the hillside.

After a little less than a mile, the trail descends into an obvious valley where a small creek runs. Just before dropping all the way to the creek, look right for a faint path. This unmarked trail is the path to the arches. Follow it about 0.1 mile—the path will drop to the creek, crossing and recrossing it, and at times the creekbed itself will be the path, so be careful not to crush any plants—before rising a last pitch to the head of the ravine and the very obvious entrance to the limestone Powder Mill Arch, carved out by eons of running water (N37° 52.011' W83° 41.125'). Notice the change in air temperature inside the arch. Go to the back right side of the arch, and you'll see a wedge in the rock with a sky hole: this is Wolf Pen Arch.

To continue the hike, head back to the main trail, then go right, crossing the creek and climbing briefly. From here to the end of the hike, the trail climbs more aggressively at times. Along the way, watch on the right side for a deep sinkhole, but *stay away from the edge*. Cell reception is spotty here, and there's no real way to call for a rescue.

At the end of the official 2.2-mile trail, you'll reach Hatton Ridge Road, a primitive doubletrack gravel road overgrown with plants. When the leaves are down, you will have great views over the Cumberland Plateau. This ridge is home to a unique plant community of white pines and eastern hemlocks, as well as red maples, yellow poplars, and sassafras, among others. Return the way you came.

Directions

From Exit 33 off Bert T. Combs Mountain Parkway, turn left on KY 11 for 0.1 mile to the intersection, then go left 1.5 miles on KY 11/15. Turn right on KY 77, which will take you through the Nada Tunnel and over the Red River, for 4.3 miles. On the far side of the steel bridge, turn left on Forest Service Road 23 and follow this paved but sometimes narrow road for 2.5 miles. At a sign for Indian Creek, turn right on FS 9/Indian Creek Road, a potholed but passable dirt road, for 1.2 miles. Just after the bridge over Indian Creek, go left at the junction and continue on FS 9A for 0.7 mile; park at a small turnout beside a metal garbage can and the sign for Powdermill Branch Trail.

28 White's Branch Arch

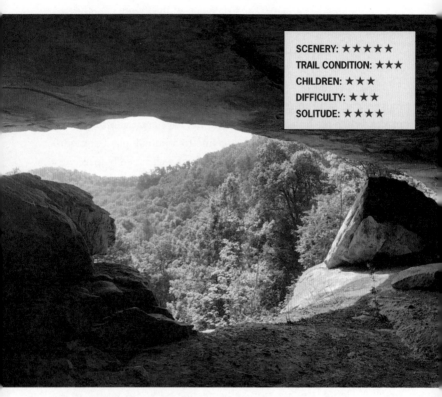

TAKE A MOMENT TO ENJOY THE VIEW FROM WHITE'S BRANCH ARCH.

> **SCENERY:** ★★★★★
> **TRAIL CONDITION:** ★★★
> **CHILDREN:** ★★★
> **DIFFICULTY:** ★★★
> **SOLITUDE:** ★★★★

GPS TRAILHEAD COORDINATES: *Hemlock Lodge parking lot* N37° 46.547' W83° 40.828'

DISTANCE & CONFIGURATION: 5.8-mile out-and-back

HIGHLIGHTS: Wooded ridgeline and a relatively unknown but magnificent sandstone arch

HIKING TIME: 3.5 hours

ELEVATION: 874' at the trailhead, with an elevation gain of 539'

ACCESS: Day use only in the Natural Bridge State Resort Park boundary, with no overnight camping allowed and hikers required to be off the trail by sunset. Outside the park boundary, camping is permitted. No dogs are allowed on trails in Natural Bridge State Resort Park.

MAPS: USGS *Slade;* Natural Bridge State Resort Park Trail Guide; USFS *Red River Gorge Geological Area*

FACILITIES: Restrooms in Hemlock Lodge

WHEELCHAIR ACCESS: None

COMMENTS: Dangerous cliffs are present and should be avoided, especially by children.

CONTACTS: Natural Bridge State Resort Park: 606-663-2214 or 800-325-1710, parks .ky.gov/parks/resortparks/natural-bridge; Kentucky State Nature Preserves Commission: 502-782-7839, eec.ky.gov/Nature-Preserves/Locations/Pages/Natural-Bridge.aspx

Overview

Natural Bridge State Resort Park—and in particular, the Natural Bridge arch—is one of the most heavily visited places in the state of Kentucky. Yet beyond the arch lies the Natural Bridge State Park Nature Preserve, more than 1,000 acres of woodlands that host the rare and federally endangered Virginia big-eared bat as well as the Hood Branch watershed, with its diverse microinvertebrate communities. Here in this backcountry you'll find the route to the lesser-known White's Branch Arch, clearly detailed on the USFS Red River Gorge map, and located along the famous Sheltowee Trace. This sandstone arch is well worth visiting, especially in the spring when migrating warblers flit among the trees and pink lady's slipper orchids dot the ridgeline.

Route Details

From the signboard at the end of the Hemlock Lodge parking area, follow the paved path past the beginning of the Original Trail to the Balanced Rock Trail on the right—also known as the Sheltowee Trace, and blazed with white turtles along the trail. Climb the limestone stairway and, at the top, turn sharply left past a large, fenced-off cave. Climb again, and at the 0.2-mile mark you'll pass Balanced Rock, one of the park's main geological attractions.

The next 0.5 mile climbs steadily and follows a ridge (beware of the cliffs) to a trail junction. If it's not crowded, head right (roughly north) to take a break and enjoy the view from Natural Bridge. Otherwise, note the big wooden sign indicating the Sand Gap Trail—this is the Sheltowee Trace, which you'll follow to White's Branch Arch.

White's Branch Arch

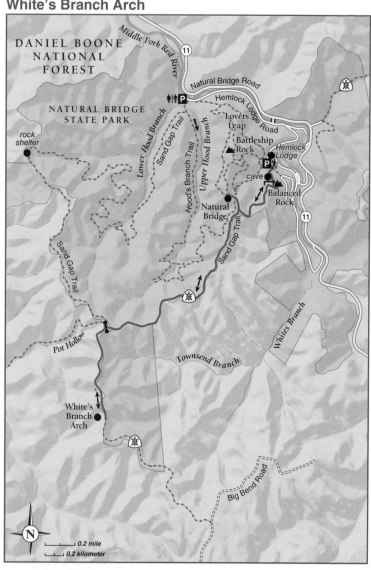

DANIEL BOONE
NATIONAL
FOREST

Middle Fork Red River

NATURAL BRIDGE
STATE PARK

Natural Bridge Road

Hemlock Lodge Road

Lovers
Leap

Battleship
Rock

Hemlock
Lodge

rock
shelter

Lower Hood Branch

Sand Gap Trail

Hood's Branch Trail

Upper Hood Branch

cave

Balanced
Rock

Natural
Bridge

Sand Gap Trail

Sand Gap Trail

Pot Hollow

Townsend Branch

Whites Branch

White's
Branch
Arch

Big Bend Road

N

0.2 mile
0.2 kilometer

Follow the Sand Gap Trail 1.6 miles along the wooded ridge to a junction with a gate. The hike continues on the other side of that gate, a continuation of the Sheltowee Trace; do not take the trail to the right, which is the continuation of the Sand Gap Trail. From here, you officially leave the state park and enter the national forest.

Follow an abandoned road for 0.6 mile. It's a rough trek in places, with plenty of exposed rock—take care when the trail is wet. You will know you are in the right place when you reach The Narrows, with drop-offs on either side of the trail and an expansive view (N37° 45.157' W83° 42.043'). At this point, you are standing on top of White's Branch Arch.

To see the arch will require a bit of scrambling. At The Narrows, look for an unmarked path on the right (west) side of the trail. Descend south along this trail, which switchbacks down a fairly steep slope. At the crook of the trail, you'll have to descend through a crack in the rock using the rope that, as of this writing, is firmly in place. Once down the crack, follow the path that runs back toward the way you came (north), and you will come to the arch. Enjoy the panorama, and return the way you came.

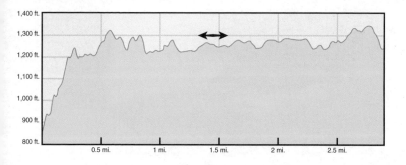

Directions

From Exit 33 off Bert T. Combs Mountain Parkway, drive south on KY 11 for 2 miles to the main entrance of Natural Bridge State Resort Park. Turn right into the entrance, and then take an immediate left, following signs for Hemlock Lodge 0.3 mile to the lot. Don't park beyond the lodge—those spaces are reserved for guests.

SUNLIGHT FILTERS THROUGH WHITE'S BRANCH ARCH.

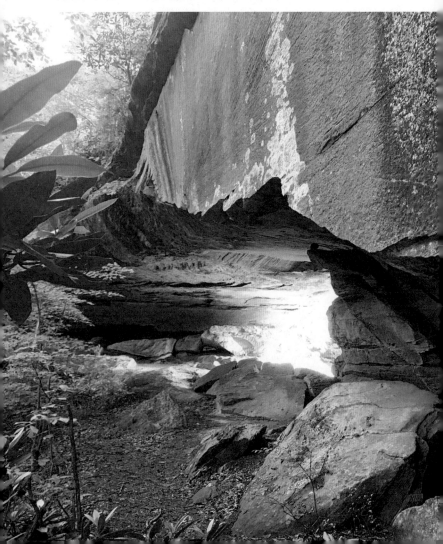

APPENDIXES & INDEX

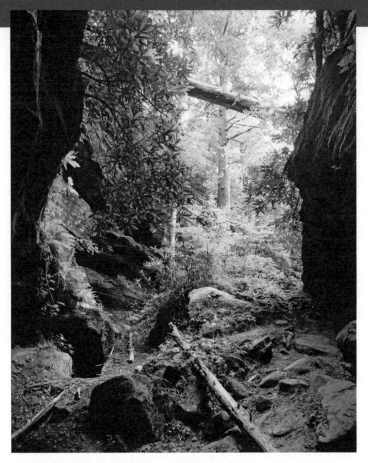

LUSH MIXED MESOPHYTIC FORESTS COVER MUCH OF THE RED RIVER GORGE.

APPENDIX A: OUTDOOR RETAILERS 174

APPENDIX B: HIKING CLUBS 176

APPENDIX C: STATE AND FEDERAL AGENCIES 177

INDEX 179

ABOUT THE AUTHOR 187

Appendix A:
Outdoor Retailers

Because of their proximity to the Red River Gorge area, Louisville, Lexington, and the Cincinnati area offer an abundance of resources for gear, maps, and other essentials.

Louisville Area

DICK'S SPORTING GOODS
dickssportinggoods.com
7900 Shelbyville Rd.
Louisville, KY 40222
502-420-6400

3500 South Hurstbourne Pkwy.
Louisville, KY 40299
502-499-9029

3555 Springhurst Blvd.
Louisville, KY 40241
502-429-0776

QUEST OUTDOORS
questoutdoors.com
4600 Shelbyville Rd.
Louisville, KY 40207
502-290-4589

Lexington Area

DICK'S SPORTING GOODS
dickssportinggoods.com
3645 Nicholasville Rd.
Lexington, KY 40503
859-273-1642

1968 Pavilion Way
Lexington, KY 40509
859-264-8800

J&H OUTDOORS STORE
jhoutdoors.com
189 Moore Dr.
Lexington, KY 40503
859-278-0730

Cincinnati/Florence Area

BENCHMARK OUTDOOR OUTFITTERS
benchmarkoutfitter.com
9525 Kenwood Rd.
Cincinnati, OH 45242
513-791-9453

DICK'S SPORTING GOODS
dickssportinggoods.com
10180 Colerain Ave.
Cincinnati, OH 45251
513-370-5022

650 Eastgate South Dr.
Cincinnati, OH 45245
513-752-5525

7800 Montgomery Rd. #275
Cincinnati, OH 45236
513-370-5024

5555 Glenway Ave.
Cincinnati, OH 45238
513-347-7570

DICK'S SPORTING GOODS (cont.)
1336 Hansel Ave., Suite 200
Florence, KY 41042
859-283-2702

GREAT MIAMI OUTFITTERS
greatmiamioutfitters.com
101 E. Alex-Bell Rd., #140
Dayton, OH 45459
937-938-5009

REI
rei.com/stores/cincinnati.html
2643 Edmondson Rd.
Cincinnati, OH 45209
513-924-1938

ALMOST 20 MILES OF THE RED RIVER ARE DESIGNATED AS A NATIONAL WILD AND SCENIC RIVER.

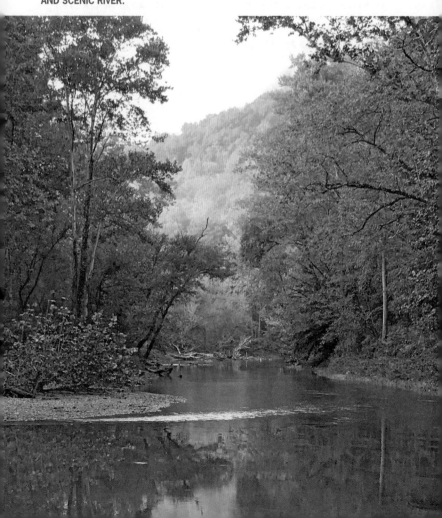

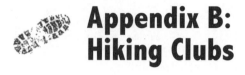

Appendix B: Hiking Clubs

Hiking clubs are a great way to get out and make friends. Plus, you can learn a lot about the Red River Gorge from some of the locals who lead these trips.

Louisville Area

LOUISVILLE HIKING CLUB MEETUP
meetup.com/LouisvilleHikingClub

KENTUCKY TRAILS ASSOCIATION
facebook.com/KentuckyTrail

Lexington Area

HIKERS OF THE BLUEGRASS
meetup.com/bluegrass-hikers

Cincinnati Area

THE MIAMI GROUP SIERRA CLUB
miamigroup.org/hiking

TRI-STATE HIKING CLUB
tristatehikingclub.com

Appendix C: State and Federal Agencies

Here is a complete list of the various management agencies for the areas of the Red River Gorge covered in this guide.

Daniel Boone National Forest
fs.usda.gov/dbnf
1700 Bypass Rd.
Winchester, KY 40391
859-745-3100

Gladie Cultural-Environmental Learning Center
tinyurl.com/gladie
3451 Sky Bridge Rd.
Stanton, KY 40380
606-663-8100

Natural Bridge State Resort Park
parks.ky.gov/parks/resortparks/natural-bridge
2135 Natural Bridge Rd.
Slade, KY 40376
606-663-2214

Natural Bridge State Park Nature Preserve
eec.ky.gov/Nature-Preserves/Locations/Pages/Natural-Bridge.aspx
300 Sower Blvd.
Frankfort, KY 40601

Index

A

Access (hike profile), 13
Adena Arch, 107
agencies, state and federal, 177
Angel Windows, 5, 32–35
animal regulations, 27
animals
    encounters with, 29
    and plants, 21–24
arches, best hikes for, xi
audio device regulations, 27
Auxier Branch Trail, 53
Auxier Ridge, 30, 41–45

B

backcountry permits, 13
backpacking, best hikes for, xi
Balanced Rock, 9, 137–141, 169
Balanced Rock Trail, 151
bats, 24
Battleship Rock, 156
Battleship Rock Trail, 139, 141,
    155, 156, 157
bears, 21
Benchmark Outdoor Outfitters,
    174
Berry, Wendell, ix
Bison Way Loop, Sheltowee Trace,
    105–109
Bison Way Trail, 111
black bears, 21
black flies, 22
book
    about this, 1–5
    how to use this, 9–14
Boone, Daniel, 4, 47, 108, 161
boots, hiking, 17
Buck Trail, 62, 65
business activity regulations, 27

C

campfire regulations, 25–26
camping regulations, 26
cell phones, 19
children. *See* kids
Chimney Top Creek, 61, 83
Chimney Top Rock, 6, 36–40
Cliff Trail, 85–89
Clifty Wilderness, 1, 3, 4, 7, 111
    hikes, 104–135
climbing precautions, 29
clothing, 16–17
Cloud Splitter Rock, 107, 109
clubs, hiking, 176
Comments (hike profile), 14
Contacts (hike profile), 14
copperhead, coral, cottonmouth
    snakes, 23
Courthouse Rock, 6, 41–45
Creation Falls, 71, 120

D

D. Boon Hut, 46–49
D. Boon Hut Trail, 76
Daniel Boone National Forest, x, 6,
    13, 101, 140, 176
Devil's Canyon, 91, 93
Devil's Gulch, 155
Devil's Gulch Trail, 157
Dick's Sporting Goods, 174–175
difficulty, star ratings, 11
Directions (hike description), 14
Distance & Configuration
    (hike profile), 12
Dog Fork, 119
dogs, 29
Double Arch, 2, 6, 50–54
Douglas, U.S. Supreme Court
    Justice William O., ix

drinking water, 15–16, 18

E

Elevation (hike profile), 13
elevation profiles, 10
etiquette, trail, 28–29

F

Facilities (hike profile), 14
Fat Man's Misery, 140, 156
fauna and flora, 21–24
federal and state agencies, 177
fee area regulations, 26
fireworks, firearm regulations, 28
first aid kits, 18–19
flora and fauna, 21–24

G

gear, essential, 17–18
geology, best hikes for, xi
giardia parasites, 16
Gladie Cabin, 114
Gladie Creek, 7, 111, 113, 114
Gladie Cultural-Environmental
   Learning Center, 13, 107, 176
GPS trailhead coordinates, 12–14
GPS units, 10
Grays Arch, 2, 6, 8, 55–58
Grays Arch Trail, 47, 76
Greasy Branch, 108–109
Great Miami Outfitters, 175
gun regulations, 28

H

Half Moon Arch, 36–40
heat exhaustion, heatstroke, 20
Hell's Kitchen, 7, 117, 119, 133
Hemlock Lodge, 141, 172
Henson's Arch Trail, 145
Henson's Cave Arch, 142–146
Hidden Arch, 59–63
Highlights (hike profile), 13

Hikers of the Bluegrass, 176
hikes
   See also specific trail
   in Clifty Wilderness, 104–135
   in Natural Bridge State Resort
      Park, 136–157
   profiles generally, 10–11
   recommended, xi–xii
   in Red River Gorge Geological
      Area, 31–103
hiking
   clothing, 16–17
   clubs, 176
   essential gear, 17–18
   first aid kits, 18–19
   general safety, 19–21
   night, 30
   shoes, boots, 17
   tips on enjoying, 29–30
   trail etiquette, 28–29
Hiking Time (hike profile), 13
Hill, Sean Patrick, 187
Hood's Branch Trail, 147, 150
Hood's Branch—Sand Gap Loop,
   147–152
hunting, 24
hypothermia, hyperthermia, 20

I

Indian Arch, 2, 81, 107, 108
Indian Creek, 166
Indian Staircase, the, 81, 82, 83,
   107, 108
insects, 22–23

J

J&H Outdoors Store, 174

K

Kentucky Trails Association, 175
kids
   best hikes for, xi

hiking with, 29–30
star ratings, 11
Koomer Ridge, 59–63
Koomer Ridge Campground, 6, 13, 87
Koomer Ridge Trail, 62, 65
KY Arch 80, 108

L
Laurel Ridge, 9
Laurel Ridge Trail, 156, 157
Left Flank Trail, 76
Lexington and Eastern Railroad, 155
Lookout Point, 155, 156
Lost Branch Trail, 82, 113
Louisville Hiking Club Meetup, 176
Lovers Leap, 155, 156, 157
Lower Hood Branch, 152
Lyme disease, 23

M
map legend, vii, 9–10
maps
  See also specific hike
  best for area, 14
  as gear, 18
  overview, legend, trail, 9–10
Martins Fork Trailhead, 76
Miami Group Sierra Club, 176
Military Wall Trail, 76
Millstone Quarry Trail, 161, 162
mosquitoes, 22
Muir, John, ix

N
Narrows, The, 171
national forest wilderness regulations, 28
Natural Bridge, 2, 8, 139, 140, 149, 151, 155

Natural Bridge State Park Nature Preserve, 167, 176
Natural Bridge State Resort Park, 1, 4, 8–9, 139, 140, 151, 155, 176
  hikes, 136–157
Needle's Eye, 157
nettles, stinging, 23
night hiking, 30

O
Original Trail, 8, 139, 141, 153–157
Osborne Bend Loop, Sheltowee Trace, 110–114
Osborne Bend Trail, 113–114
Oscar Geralds, Jr. Trail, 161, 162
outdoor retailers, 174–175
Overview (hike description), 14
overview maps, 9–10

P
Parched Corn Creek, 33, 97
permits, backcountry, 13
pet regulations, 27
Pilot Knob, 161
Pilot Knob State Nature Preserve, 159–162
Pinch-Em-Tight Ridge, 64–67
Pinch-Em-Tight Trail, 63, 77, 83
plants and animals, 21–24
poison ivy, oak, 22
Powdermill Arch, 166
Powdermill Branch Trail, 163–167
precipitation, average monthly, 15
Princess Arch, 36–40
profiles, hike, 10–11
property regulations, 26–27
public behavior regulations, 27

Q
Quest Outdoors, 174

R
rain, average monthly, 15
raingear, 17
ratings, star, 11
rattlesnakes, 23
recommended hikes, xi–xii
Red River, 6, 30, 81, 83, 111, 114
Red River Gorge
  described, ix–x, 1–5
  geological area, 6–7
  regulations, 24–28
  tips on enjoying hiking in,
    29–30
  weather, 15
Red River Gorge Geological Area,
  1, 6–7
  hikes, 31–103
regulations, 24–28
REI outfitters, 175
retailers, outdoor, 174–175
Rock Bridge Arch, 68–72, 119
Rock Bridge Recreation Area, 133,
  134
Rock Bridge Trail, 119
Rock Garden, the, 9
Rock Garden Trail, 137–141
Rough Trail, 4, 6, 58, 62, 65, 73–78
Route Details (hike description), 14
Rush Ridge Trail, 58

S
safety, general, 2–3, 19–21
Sage Point Trail, 161, 162
Sal Branch, 114
Salt Fork, 111, 113
Sand Gap Loop, Hood's Branch,
  147–152
Sand Gap Trail, 9, 140, 150, 169,
  171
sandstone arches, x
sanitation regulations, 24–25
Sawyer, Diane, ix

scenery, star ratings, 11
scenic creeks, best hikes for, xi
seasons to visit, 3–4, 15
seclusion, best hikes for, xi
Sheltowee Trace, 1, 4, 9, 62–63,
  77, 79–84, 99, 139, 150, 169
  Bison Way Loop, 105–109
  Osborne Bend Loop, 110–114
shoes, hiking, 17
Signature Rock, 63, 81, 83
Silvermine Arch, 2, 85–89
Sky Bridge, 6, 90–93
Slade USGS topographic map, 14
snakes, 23
solitude, star ratings, 11
Sons Branch, 118, 126
star ratings, 11
state and federal agencies, 177
stinging nettles, 23
Suspension Bridge Trailhead, 109
Swift Camp Creek, 7, 71, 91
  Swift Camp Creek Trail, 71,
    115–120, 134
  Wildcat Loop, 121–126

T
temperatures, average monthly, 15
ticks, 23
Timmons Arch, 124
Tower Rock, 127–130
trail condition, star ratings, 11
trail etiquette, 28–29
trail maps, 10
trailhead coordinates, GPS, 12–14
Tri-State Hiking Club, 176
Turtle Back Arch, 7, 131–135

U
Unforeseen Wilderness, The (Berry),
  ix
Upper Hood Branch, 150
Upper Hood Branch Loop, 151

V

vehicle regulations, 25
views, best hikes for, xii
Virginia big-eared bats, 24
Virginia pines, xii

W

water, drinking, 15–16, 18
weather, 15
Wheelchair Access (hike profile), 14
whistles, 20
white-haired goldenrod, 24

White's Branch Arch, 168–172
Whittleton Arch, 2, 94–97, 98–103, 143
Whittleton Branch, 99, 143
Whittleton Branch Trail, 143
Whittleton Campground, 101, 103, 143, 145
Whittleton Fork, 143
Wildcat Creek, 118, 124, 125
Wildcat Trail, 119, 124
wildflowers, best hikes for, xii
Wolf Pen Arch, 166, 167

Check out this great title from
Menasha Ridge Press!

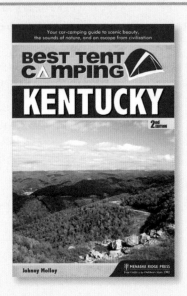

Best Tent Camping: Kentucky

Johnny Molloy
ISBN: 978-1-63404-004-4
$15.95, 2nd Edition

6 x 9, paperback
192 pages
maps and photos

Best Tent Camping: Kentucky leads you to the best tent-camping destinations within the Bluegrass State, describing not only the campgrounds themselves, but also the fun outdoorsy activities nearby. The book uses a rating system, which includes campground privacy, security, beauty, quiet, and cleanliness, and gives inside tips on how to enjoy each particular destination from your chosen campground. It also details prices, opening and closing dates, websites, and other information that will help you utilize your precious time to the fullest and make the most of your Kentucky tent-camping experience.

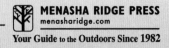

MENASHA RIDGE PRESS
menasharidge.com

Your Guide to the Outdoors Since 1982

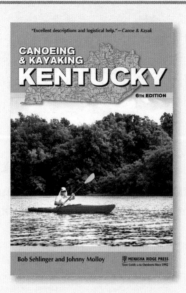
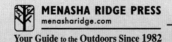

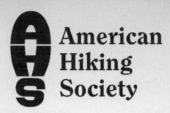

American Hiking Society

PROTECT THE PLACES YOU LOVE TO HIKE.

Become a member today and
take $5 off using the code **Hike5**.

AmericanHiking.org/join

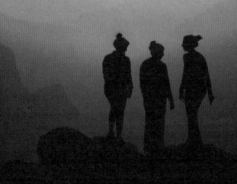

American Hiking Society is the only
national nonprofit organization dedicated
to empowering all to enjoy, share, and
preserve the hiking experience

© Karl Magnuson / kmagnuson.com

About the Author

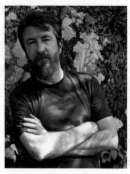

SEAN PATRICK HILL lives in Louisville, Kentucky, where he spends time with his daughter, practices photography, and writes. As a hiker and backpacker, he has walked trails across the country, from the Pacific Crest Trail to the Appalachian Trail, including rambles in the Grand Canyon, the Delaware Water Gap, Yosemite National Park, the Rocky Mountains, the Olympic Peninsula, and the Oregon Cascades. In Kentucky, he tends to stick to the Bernheim Arboretum and Research Forest (where he volunteers as a trail ranger) and the Jefferson Memorial Forest, though he will on occasion ramble as far as Pine Mountain, the Cumberland Gap, and, of course, the Red River Gorge.

DEAR CUSTOMERS AND FRIENDS,

SUPPORTING YOUR INTEREST IN OUTDOOR ADVENTURE, travel, and an active lifestyle is central to our operations, from the authors we choose to the locations we detail to the way we design our books. Menasha Ridge Press was incorporated in 1982 by a group of veteran outdoorsmen and professional outfitters. For many years now, we've specialized in creating books that benefit the outdoors enthusiast.

Almost immediately, Menasha Ridge Press earned a reputation for revolutionizing outdoors- and travel-guidebook publishing. For such activities as canoeing, kayaking, hiking, backpacking, and mountain biking, we established new standards of quality that transformed the whole genre, resulting in outdoor-recreation guides of great sophistication and solid content. Menasha Ridge Press continues to be outdoor publishing's greatest innovator.

The folks at Menasha Ridge Press are as at home on a whitewater river or mountain trail as they are editing a manuscript. The books we build for you are the best they can be, because we're responding to your needs. Plus, we use and depend on them ourselves.

We look forward to seeing you on the river or the trail. If you'd like to contact us directly, visit us at menasharidge.com. We thank you for your interest in our books and the natural world around us all.

SAFE TRAVELS,

Bob Sehlinger

BOB SEHLINGER
PUBLISHER